The Other Side of

Alzheimer's,

A caregivers story

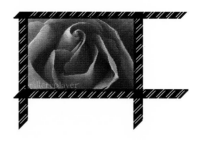

THE *OTHER* SIDE

OF

ALZHEIMER'S

A caregiver's story

Marietta A. Harris

RBMB Publishing Company/2009

San Francisco, CA

Special Thanks to:

Dr. Ken Woolridge

Shari Carver

Janice Buxton

Dorla Cummins

Carol Fairweather

Editor: Edith Gladstone

THROUGH DIFFICULTIES

...WE CONQUER

Roxie Quincy Louise Maria Harris

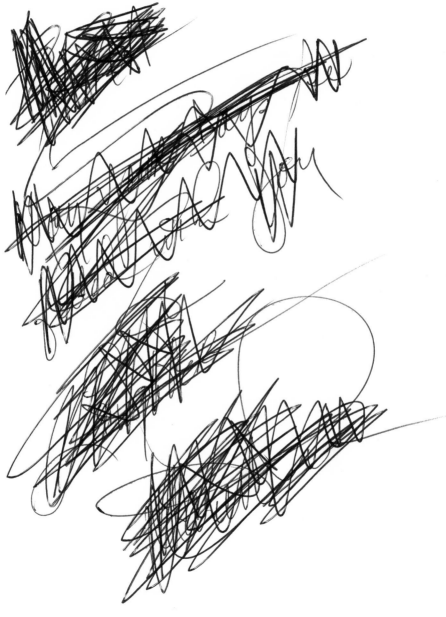

Chapter 1

It is 3:00 a.m. and I'm still awake. Moving and unpacking was more than I expected and now I can't fall asleep in my new house. Building it took almost a year. Now I'm finally here. I can't hear any noise outside, just dead silence. There are only three other houses on this block. From my bed, I can see bright stars in the sky. My heart's still racing.

It took the movers and me hours to drive here from my San Francisco apartment and another four hours to empty the truck of all my stuff. I can't believe I have so much stuff. I gave away much from my old life because I need to start anew. I can feel myself falling asleep.

I look over at the clock and it is 10:00 a.m. Before opening my eyes, I could feel the sun on my face. It is good to be alive. I am happy. I start to giggle.

My spirit is finding peace in my bright new room. Boxes are everywhere, but I don't care. It is a beautiful day. The house smells new. My bedroom is huge. I have always wanted a big house, like the one I grew up in as a child. The real estate agent kept trying to show me condominiums and small houses but I was not settling until I had the house that I wanted. I needed to have lots of rooms.

My car is in my garage. My bills are paid. I have money in the bank. Did I mention I am in my new house? My time is my time—so if I want to, I can just lie in this bed all day. But I'm overwhelmed with excitement. I haven't felt like this since I was a child, when I couldn't wait to run downstairs on Christmas morning to unwrap my presents.

I feel a sudden urge to unpack. I am home. The thought astounds me. It's been years since I have felt so happy. For years now, I've felt guilty being happy.

I fumble through a box marked clothes and find a sweat suit. Towels are right there in the box marked linen. After showering, I dress and head downstairs to make myself a cup of coffee. I maneuver past boxes to the kitchen and manage to find a cup, coffee, and sugar.

While waiting for the water to boil I see a box marked "fragile-pictures." My heart skips a beat. Momentarily, I'm saddened as memories flood through me. The sound of the boiling water brings me back to reality. The coffee is hot so I sit at the dining room table and look out at my unfinished backyard. I'm going to need a gardener. I don't do dirt.

Sipping the coffee, I realize I don't like coffee. In fact, I never liked coffee. I can't even remember why I starting drinking it. I make a mental note, Buy tea.

Unpacking some kitchen boxes, I find two sets of brand-new pots and pans. Where did these come from? Then I remember. Brian bought these for me as we planned our wedding. Brian! It's been years since I even thought of him. I hope and pray he has made a good life for himself. Box after box I unpack and place items in the kitchen cabinets. By the time I finish, most of the cabinets are full.

When I open the last kitchen box, I find Mom's tea set. She made the pieces with her very own hands. I remember her taking the pottery class. Mom was always taking classes. After each class, she would bring home a new object. She made dishes and bowls. She even made Dad an ashtray.

For her last class project, she designed and made the tea set, initialing every piece. That was over forty years ago. Mother was so proud and we were proud of her. She used it on special occasions, especially when the women of the neighborhood came over to visit.

I turn toward my huge family room. The box marked "fragile pictures" is still unopened. I know I have to unpack them but this is not going to be easy. I can do this. Wow—did I really say it aloud? I pull the box over to the dining room chair and sit down.

The top picture is our family portrait, which consisted of Dad, Mother, Daniel, and me. Mother always had a professional photographer come to the house for family pictures. She chose the colors we were to wear. I always enjoyed family pictures. We were a handsome family. If they were here with me, Dad would be examining the fixtures, water heater, and gas lines to make sure they were installed correctly. Mother would be making sure items in the kitchen cabinet were in their proper places. Daniel would be checking out the neighborhood to make sure it was safe for me. I miss them so much. I kiss their faces through the glass and put the portrait back on top of the box. I am going to have to do this some other time.

I head upstairs. I have a lifetime to unpack, so I'll take it one day at a time.

Chapter 2

Do you ever think about the words, "and they lived happily ever after"? I love stories that end that way. I am a romantic. I want to hear the music swell in the background and watch the couple look into each other's eyes, smile, and embrace with loving passion. When the screen fades to black, I just know that they will be happy for the rest of their lives. Days later, I will remember the movie and imagine that I was the girl in the story. Yes, I am a true romantic. I cry at the drop of a hat.

My name is Angie and I was born in San Francisco, California. Maria, my mother, said I was born with my eyes open. I was the firstborn, so you know what that means. Edward, my dad, spoiled me at birth. He was so proud that anybody he met received a cigar. Mother said he smiled for weeks. I was my dad's baby girl. Two years later, my brother Daniel arrived. Cigars sprouted again. He was Mommy's baby boy.

My parents were late bloomers. Dad was in his late fifties when I was born. He grew up in New Orleans, Louisiana, and had been born there in

1895. Dad was one of seven siblings, three boys, and four girls. Dad's family now lived in the San Francisco Bay Area. One of Dad's brothers lived in San Mateo and another lived in San Francisco. All of them owned their own homes.

Mother was born in Hattiesburg, Mississippi—the youngest of eight children, four boys, and four girls. Mom's brothers still lived on the farm where they all grew up. All my aunts and uncles were in their late fifties and sixties when I was born, and Mom was in her late forties. Most of us went to different churches. My uncles were Catholic, my cousins were Pentecostal, and my parents were Baptist.

My family was close, really close. After church on Sundays, we all met at my Aunt Emma's house for family dinner. She could cook any other chef under the table. All my aunts and uncles were awesome in the kitchen. Each had a cooking specialty. Dad was the gumbo king. Uncle Wilbur was the king of stews. Mother and Aunt Ollie cooked the best fried and smothered chicken. Uncle Will was the cornbread king. We ate the best homemade dinners anyone could make. The adults ate in the dining room. Children ate in the kitchen. It didn't matter to us kids because that meant we were closer to the food and got second servings faster. The house was filled with the aroma of good food. Conversations and laughter filled the air.

Growing up, we were allowed to play after church and before dinner. The house would be warm when we walked in the door. We could smell the food cooking and hear everyone laughing and talking. Homemade dinner rolls, sweet potato pie, fried and smothered chicken, greens, mashed potatoes, and ham. It was just down-home cooking. All the food was cooked from scratch. My favorite was hot water cornbread.

Two of my uncles worked for United Airlines and Dad worked for the Southern Pacific Railroad. Mother was a homemaker, but she often told us of the job she had when she first met Dad in the 1940s. She was driving a cable car and he struck up a conversation with her.

Mother had no problem with discipline. Dad, on the other hand, was the quiet type, a slow burner. When he said to stop doing something, he never raised his voice. He would quietly tell you to stop. He did this two times. Normally there wasn't a third time. I was very much in tune with Dad's moods but, unfortunately, my brother never really got the message. He would be playing and Dad would tell him to stop two times. Daniel would push the issue and suddenly there would be this hand. No matter what my brother was doing, it stopped him in his tracks.

When we became adults, we would sometimes reminisce about "the Hand." Daniel said he would go into his room, in the back of the closet, with the door closed, where Dad couldn't hear him, and talk about the "Hand of Death." I avoided many a punishment because I knew when to stop and sit down when I was told. Daniel was the runner. He did not understand the theory of the consequences of your actions. My mother would call him to come for a spanking—yes, that is what they did. He knew he deserved it, but he would tear off running around the house, up the stairs, down the hall, and into his room.

There were twenty-one rooms in our house so Mother was not running after him. She didn't move a step. She would tell him that when he returned, as he would have to do, she was going to make it worse because he ran. And I'd go to another room and cry. Not for myself, but because I knew the woman meant what she said. Daniel would get the spanking, but I would cry. Go figure!

Daniel was always getting into trouble. For some reason he wanted to be everyone's friend and sometimes his choices of friends were bad. Daniel found friends who did not live in our neighborhood. Their parents did not have the same rules in their house as we had in ours. No child ever called my dad, or any dad, by his first name.

I remember when Daniel first went to school. Emerson Elementary School was three blocks away from our house. For some reason, instead of coming directly home after school, Daniel would be an hour late. Mother reminded him that he had better be home by 3:30 since he got out of school at 3:00.

Because I was his big sister, Mother insisted I meet him after school and escort him home before Dad decided to make another brother. To my surprise, as I waited outside the school fence, Daniel came out of the door and ran the other way.

At first, I assumed he was avoiding me, but then I saw a girl running after him. Maybe this could be the reason why he was late. Sure enough, he ran the opposite direction from the house. I saw this little girl running after him. She was close on his tail and I couldn't catch them, so I called to him, but he wasn't stopping.

I decided to just go home. Sure enough, at 4:10 he came running from the opposite direction. He hit the steps two at a time, with this little girl right behind him. I was waiting there. Daniel said the girl had been running him home for several days. I explained to that girl the nature of pain and how I meant to inflict it on her if she touched my brother. She never bothered him again. Apparently, she had a real bad crush on him but he was too young to know it.

I remember Mother's face when I told her why Daniel was late. Mother held her composure so well. We were taught not to start fights, but she told my brother that he could defend himself. She further explained that he could not be the aggressor. She especially did not want him fighting girls. I remember Mother explaining this to Dad. He turned around and walked away. When he thought we couldn't hear him, he starting laughing so hard. Years later Dad and Mom would talk about that little girl and we all would laugh, especially because she was younger and smaller than Daniel. (She later became his first girlfriend. Daniel learned how to defend himself and, in some cases, defended himself too much. If he came home late, it was because he'd been chasing some girl.)

Chapter 3

The four of us lived in our big house in San Francisco's Lower Pacific Heights. When Dad purchased our house, there were only two African-American families in the neighborhood. Despite the fact that the majority of our neighbors were white, mixed, or Asian we never felt any prejudice or were treated differently. All of us children played together. Hide-and-go-seek, baseball, jacks—you name it, we played it. We had no fear of playing outside. We could play outside until it started to get dark. We went to each other's houses and obeyed each other's parents. All the moms and dads knew and respected each other.

Jim and Sally were Chinese and owned the neighborhood store. They were always nice to us kids. We played with their kids, Mia and Andrew. If we did not have enough money for candy, Sally would let us have it anyway. We were not allowed to call an adult by their first name so we called her Mrs. Sally. There was a well-known rule in our neighborhood: if another kid's mother gave you a spanking; you knew when you got home you were going to get another one from your mom. When I look back, our block was like a village. Everybody raised us. On both sides of our block, there were streetlights. When the streetlights came on, everyone knew it was time to go home. As children, we had no sense of danger. When I think about it, God really protected us because we were just dangerous when it came to making up games.

The street on our block was flat, and traffic moved in both directions. At each intersection it became one way, so you went uphill from one corner and down from the other, toward downtown. One day we found a shopping cart. Well, it offered too much temptation. We started out with one of us getting in the cart and pushing it down the street.

That excitement soon turned dull. It wasn't dangerous enough. Someone got this crazy idea to take the shopping cart and push it up the hill, halfway. One of us would get in the cart and ride down the hill. What a ride! We were all laughing and talking loud while riding down the hill with no way to stop the cart. We had no sense of danger. Of course, we hadn't taken into consideration that going down the hill we should make sure the light was green. Our only objective in life was to have fun.

Timing was critical, and only God knows how we are alive today. Amazing as it sounds, we always made the green light, missed the traffic, and no one ever fell out of the cart or broke a bone. All we suffered were a lot of scrapes and scares. That game ended when one of our mothers saw what we were doing. We heard this horrible sound of her screaming our names. She provided us with the spankings of a lifetime. In those days it wasn't uncommon to have one of your friends run up to you and proclaim, "Your mommy said come home, now." Can you remember the innocence and pure joy of being a kid?

Chapter 4

Dad worked for the Southern Pacific Railroad from 4:00 p.m. to midnight. During the day, he would devote his time to the church as the senior deacon. He was also a self-taught carpenter and a real estate broker. He would help fix up homes for members of his congregation and others. Sometimes he would buy an apartment building, fix it up, and then sell it.

Mother stayed at home, like the mom on the TV show *Leave it to Beaver.* For as long as I could remember, Mother was always home. Cooking, cleaning, sewing, knitting, and taking care of the family were her pride and joy. She was an excellent seamstress. She also knitted, crocheted, and kept our house very clean. Instead of talking bad about people, all she ever would say was, "I wish the person had a better attitude" or "How unfortunate he or she never grew up emotionally as they did physically."

Mother was also a writer. For years, she would take time during the day to sit down and write in her books. Being a Christian woman, she was writing books to help younger Christians understand how difficult it was to try to live in this world as a Christian. She was always a teacher. She taught Sunday school, BTU (that's Baptist Training Union), and children's church. Her classes were always crowded because she encouraged students to participate. She gave them challenges, which made them want to learn the subject. Mother was very active in the church mission as the pianist and teacher of a Mission Circle.

There was no slamming of doors or Dad leaving the house in a huff. I remember thinking that I sure wanted a marriage like my parents'. One day, I came home and found them in the kitchen cooking together. As I went out the door on the way to my room, Dad gently patted Mother on the behind. I could hear her giggle. Then there were times when she would pass by him and squeeze his upper arm. He'd never change the look on his face but his eyes glowed, even through his glasses.

They did have days when they were angry with each other. I remember them sitting in the living room, Dad reading his paper and Mother knitting and neither one of them saying a word. Or sometimes they would sit and talk for hours, even after we were in bed. Daniel and I knew that we had better not get involved. Nevertheless, their motto was they would never go to bed angry. By the next morning; they were back to talking to each other again.

Summers were great. Either we went to our ranch in Santa Rosa or we visited my grandmother, Mother's mom, in Mississippi. On the way there, Mother explained that life in Mississippi was different from life in San Francisco. Remember, this was in the 1950s and 60s. We already knew how to address adults with Yes, ma'am, or No, sir, because that was how we were raised. I wasn't sure why the rest rooms in Hattiesburg were labeled "white" and "colored." We obeyed Mother and didn't have any problems.

When I was born, it was fashionable to be called "Negro" and my parents accepted that word. In the 60s, the word changed to "Black." Well, this did not set very well in our house, especially since both my parents grew up in the South. To them it was too harsh of a word to accept. Frankly, if you called Daddy *Black*, he would take great offense and explain that his preference was Negro and he was not some Black man. In the late 80s and early 90s, we were known as "Afro-Americans." My parents could not understand why our race could not decide on what we are. Daddy always said, "If you have to keep changing your name, then you'll never be what you really are and that's just a dark skin American."

We were not poor, nor were we rich. I guess you could say we were middle class. Our twenty-one-room house was marvelous. Daniel and I had our own bedrooms and bathrooms. Dad was older than the other fathers, but he was well respected and admired by them. He was intelligent, hardworking, and a Christian man. He had high morals and treated others with dignity and respect. Everyone who knew him treated him with dignity and respect.

Both my parents were readers. So there was a large selection of books in our library. I enjoyed reading a book a week and spent many days studying and reading in the library.

Daniel and I attended good public schools, had nice clothes, and all the other amenities we wanted. My parents were involved with our education and always went to parent-teacher meetings. Daniel and I were privileged in many ways, but not to the point of being egotistical or arrogant. As I said, Dad was born in New Orleans and Mother was from Hattiesburg, Mississippi. They both believed in raising us in the "traditional way." That meant spankings. Being spanked didn't kill us. What it did was emphasize our errors in a more memorable manner. It provided boundaries. Some may say it's cruel, but neither Daniel nor I ever had problems with the law. And I do not understand "time out." I'm not sure, what does it teach? From what I see, children today need something stronger than time out. It just provides them time to figure out how not to get caught the next time. Sorry, I will leave that subject alone.

Chapter 5

Daddy enjoyed buying and selling property. From the earliest time I can remember, Daddy was always involved in real estate. He was also a Senior Deacon at his church. Even though he did not go to work until 4:00 p.m., he ate breakfast and left the house, wearing a suit. There was never a day that Dad was not in a suit, tie, and fedora hat.

Dad loved fixing things around the house and helping other people. I remember when I was seven or eight, I asked him to build me a tree house in the backyard,—you know the kind of tree house where you climb up on a makeshift ladder and pretend you are looking over the yard. Well, by the time he was finished, Dad had built a small two-story house with electricity, drywall, and everything. He used the lower level to store his tools. The second floor was a large room with windows and a door that locked. There was a walkway between the main house and the small house. Later, when I grew up and wanted a place of my own, I moved to the tree house. It had a separate entrance through the garden.

Mother was a wonderful lady, and I emphasize Lady. In all her years, whether or not I lived with her, I never saw Mother without her hair coiffed, wearing a nice dress, and an apron. She was the caretaker of the house. Mother was always up before anyone else and the last to go to bed. Waking up and smelling her breakfast was such a thrill. We had eggs, toast, grits or oatmeal and orange juice. Saturdays, if she felt like it, she would make homemade biscuits. We never left home without eating breakfast. I was never really an everyday breakfast person. A glass of orange juice and toast was all I ever wanted.

Cooking was Mother's pride and joy, along with keeping the house clean. She was a deaconess at her church and highly respected. She carried herself with such dignity. She was a private woman. Mother would never be on the telephone gossiping about anyone. I remember Dad telling her that since the house was so large she should hire someone to help. Mother cleaned the house before the housekeeper arrived, then they would have the rest of the day to enjoy drinking coffee, sewing, or going shopping. Dad tried to explain to her that

Mildred was not hired to be her companion. She just laughed and walked away. Sometimes she would actually let Mildred clean the windows or polish the silverware. Mother was like that; she enjoyed being a homemaker.

My parents did not drink, curse, or fight. I can't remember ever hearing a cross word between them. If there were differences, they kept it to themselves. Dad loved to smoke cigars. The only time he would smoke was after dinner. At dinner, the family sat down together and enjoyed each other's company. We would talk about problems at school, plan a weekend, or just have funny conversations. After dinner the table was cleared, I washed dishes, Daniel would take out the trash, and we would all go into the living room. My parents enjoyed classical music and insisted that this was what I would learn. And since I was taking lessons, I always had to play something.

While I played, Mother would knit or crochet. Dad and Daniel would sit and listen. In the wintertime, Dad would light a fire in the dining room while we ate. Then he'd light a fire in the living room after dinner. Eventually we would pull out the Scrabble game and play until it was time for Daniel and me to go to bed. It was the best time of my life.

Our parents taught us how to behave, and that wisdom carried us throughout our lives. We never developed the "I'm better than you" attitude. Love permeated our house, and hugs and kisses were mandatory. The rules of the house were not made to be broken.

It was a ritual in our house for Mother to cook Monday through Friday and Sunday. Saturday was Dad's day to cook. The man could cook! Like I said, he was from N'oleans, and just knowing Dad was going to cook on Saturdays was always exciting. Not to take away from Mother's cooking, but Dad could really cook some great meals. We never knew what he might fix. The man could cook gumbo. I mean Gumbo that made you not use a napkin but lick your fingers, as my mother would say, "like you was born in the country." Red beans and rice and oh my dad's Jambalaya. Sometimes he would have a relative send crawfish, shrimp, and seasoning from home.

Since my parents were religious, family

prayers and Bible study, in our house was required on Saturday nights. They were not fanatics but strong believers. I am glad for that, because my faith has carried me through life up until this present moment. Some of the situations and people I have had to deal with in my life really tested my faith. If I wasn't a Christian, I probably would have beaten the hell out of somebody by now.

Chapter 6

My godmother, Mrs. Lillie Gordon, lived ten blocks from our house. My parents had lived in one of her apartments when got they married, so they were close friends with her and her husband, Berry. I called her Mother Gordon. She and Berry owned a very large building with a store under it, and they didn't work. She was always busy so she didn't come to our house too often.

When Mother Gordon and her husband came to dinner, especially if she was taking me somewhere, she always dressed in expensive clothes and wore a fur. I especially loved the way she carried herself. On special occasions, she would bring a gift for Daniel as well as me. I never knew why Daniel didn't have a godmother. (People would always stare when she and Mother went downtown, because both women knew how to dress.) Occasionally, she would come by the house and take me to the Ocean Beach Amusement Park. Since Mother Gordon didn't drive, either Dad would drive us or we would take the bus. (I rode the bus only with Mother Gordon, so for me it was an adventure, watching different people get on and off.)

Ocean Beach was famous in San Francisco. It was like a theme park except it had booths and rides, a scary house, and food. . Everyone went to Ocean Beach either to walk around on the beach or enjoy the carnival-like activities. I remember the dime games where you had to throw a dime and land it on a saucer to win a prize. There was also a game using three knitting hoops. The object of the game was to get at least one hoop around a stuffed animal. At the entrance to the scary house there was a ten-foot wooden "clown lady," Laughing Sal. Her hands and head moved and she laughed very loud.

Mother Gordon started taking me there when I was five years old. The first time I saw Laughing Sal, she was the scariest thing I had ever seen. As I grew up, my terror eased but she was still scary. Mother Gordon gave me money to ride as many rides as I wanted. I always came home with stuffed toys and gifts for my brother. Sometimes Mother Gordon took me to museums, plays, the ballet, and the opera. I always enjoyed our outings. She taught me to appreciate the arts. Or sometimes

Dad and Mom would take us to an opera or ballet. The *Nutcracker Suite* was my favorite. It was the best time of my life.

Mother Gordon opened up a bank account for my college education when I was born, but I didn't know about it. She kept depositing money in my account even after I graduated. She never stopped giving me gifts and money as I grew up. Even though Daniel didn't have a godmother, my parents made sure that he was never lacking for anything.

Chapter 7

When he was five years old, Daniel started taking music lessons, as I did at the same age. My instrument was the piano. My brother's instrument of choice was the clarinet. He fought it with all his might and won his battle of not wanting to play an instrument because he simply forgot everything he was taught, lesson-by-lesson. I loved the challenge and thirsted for more. I could remember anything and everything I was taught (apparently I had a musical photographic memory).

Things were so easy for me that when the teacher came for my lessons, I had learned the old one and would have already taught myself the next lesson or two. This was a BIG mistake, because my eagerness led my parents to add more instruments for me. The first were the Hammond and pipe organ Then it was the violin. (I still didn't "get it.") It seemed every instrument my music teachers suggested, my parents agreed to add it to my repertoire. Now, I had piano lessons on Monday, organ lessons on Wednesday, and violin lessons on Friday. Did I forget to mention that there was also voice lessons and ballet? I quickly passed the scales and progressed to Mozart and Beethoven. I must admit I love Beethoven. I'd play for hours dreaming of what he must have been feeling at the time he wrote the piece I'd be playing. Of course, with all these lessons, you can imagine what a dork I was. I finally realized this could go on forever.

My playtime with other kids got shorter and shorter. But if your mother was like mine, you heard statements like having these skills will help you some day. Right! I even wanted my brother to join me in the quest to play every instrument under the sun, but he was too busy playing baseball. I think about her words now and I appreciate her love, patience, and fortitude. I know this: if I can't find a regular job, I can find a job as a musician. I've got skills.

Having to take all these lessons meant Mother needed to learn how to drive. I remember them going out one evening when Dad was going to teach her. Apparently, it didn't go so well, because the next thing we knew she called the driving school and was taking driving lessons in the afternoons. Once she'd completed the course, Dad bought her a car. He was happy because now he didn't have to come home and chauffeur us around anymore. She and I were on the road! Many times, we would come home only to find that he and Daniel had gone somewhere. Dad signed Daniel up to play baseball after school so he wasn't getting out of having to do some activity after school.

Chapter 8

I remember so many days coming home to find that Mother had either bought or made me a new dress. She loved to sew and knit. Regularly, she would sew dresses or knit hats and scarves for ladies in the church who were not able to buy new clothes. Many a day I would come home only to find some of the ladies trying on a dress Mother made. She had the biggest heart. In fact, both my parents were givers.

Remember what it felt like to take a hot bath and get into bed where your sheets smelled so fresh? It was especially nice because Mother would let the sheets dry on a clothesline (eventually we got a washer and dryer). When we came home from school, dinner was always prepared; the house was always, always clean. I remember coming home, opening the front door and the whole house smelled of home cooking. Sometimes she would try new dishes like a tuna casserole.

Saturdays were special. Some Saturday mornings, we'd wake up to the smell of homemade biscuits. Dad would take Daniel with him and they would go to someone's house to build stairs, do some plumbing work, or just help someone with their house. Dad would give him money so Daniel would learn how to earn a living like a man. Dad would even help fix their roof. Mother and I got dressed to go downtown. In those days, going downtown was always an event. Everyone dressed up to go downtown.

Mother would put on her everyday hat, with purse, gloves, and a little fox on her shoulder (as Mother taught me, a lady was not dressed unless she wore gloves, hat, and a little fur to go downtown). Women took pride in their dress, in their walk and their talk. Talking loud would get me in trouble. Of course, wearing pants wasn't an option in our house. Occasionally I was allowed to wear pants in the backyard and as I got older, I could wear them while playing with the other children.

There were times when Mother and I were the best of friends. Then there were times when we challenged each other's nerves, as all mothers and daughters do. I was trying to grow up and be independent, but Mother still treated me like her little girl. And her wisdom always helped to pull us back together again. Mother taught me how to be a real woman.

I learned how to be strong, yet flexible, caring but not overbearing, and loving but not foolish. She taught me to respect myself. When you respect yourself, then you know how to treat others. You also know how you should be treated. It is disturbing to me to hear women discuss being physically or verbally abused, and still stay in the relationships for years. I suppose I might be in a similar situation except for those talks with Mother. I am so grateful for them today.

My most embarrassing talk with Mother was about the opposite sex. I was thirteen years old and was a size 36B and my special time started. Mother made it an "event." On that Thursday, I came home to find her dressed, coat in hand waiting for me. She proclaimed that it was my day and that we were going out to dinner, just the two of us. As she drove to the restaurant, the joy I felt was uncontrollable. She asked me where I wanted to go and I said Mel's Drive-In on Geary Boulevard—the restaurant Spencer Tracy and Katherine Hepburn went to in the movie *Guess Who's Coming to Dinner*. I liked it because the waitresses wore skates. They would skate up to your car window and take your order.

We went inside and sat in a booth. I ordered a cheeseburger, fries, and a root beer float. After we finished, she starting telling me about how special I was and how now that I was growing up I needed to know a few things. I will remember that talk until I die. My eyes must have been bigger than half dollars because I knew I was going to learn about sex. Well, when she finished, I knew sex was not an option for me until I got married.

Years later, Mother confessed that Dad had seen me playing outside and decided I needed the talk as soon as possible. I didn't understand why all the boys, white and Black, wanted to talk to me or why their eyes glowed when I wore a sweater. I found out Daddy had quizzed Mother that night, making sure she had stressed the "keep your dress down," "sit with your knees closed," and "wear your bra at all times." And we all laughed about how Dad was so protective. From that day, I would catch Dad frequently looking out the window to make sure I was okay.

Mother talked to me about my emotions and

how she knew there would be times when, because my body was developing, I might think I was a woman. Well, she reminded me, there was only one woman in the house, and I was looking at her. She shared with me what a joy it is to be a woman, and how precious it is to know I could bring forth life. After she said that, she sat back in her chair, looking at me with loving eyes, and continued her stern speech. She said if I brought forth a child, I had better be married, with a ring on my finger, living in my own house and with a husband.

After our talk, I was so cautious when holding hands with a boy that kissing was almost out of the question. She firmly scared the hell out of me. And that day left me with a real closeness with her.

We were women, Black women, and proud of it. She reminded me that as a Black woman I didn't need, "a man" to take care of me or to make me whole. I was going to get a good education, whether I wanted to or not and in time, the Lord would provide me with a husband. That motivated me. Suddenly I knew that was what my parents had. I lived with them all those years and I watched

Mother and Dad. However, it was on that day I finally realized what they had. It was a sharing experience.

Chapter 9

On my sixteenth birthday, Dad bought me my own car. My classmates teased me, saying I was spoiled but I really didn't have the time to be concerned about their jealousy. To me the car was no big deal. I was studying to be a concert pianist so I had piano lessons to take. I was good enough to play in the San Francisco Youth Symphony as first violinist. I really did enjoy playing the violin even though it required me to have short nails. After high school my heart really wasn't in it, and so I and focused more on the piano. My parents realized Daniel's real talent was painting and they allowed him to take classes. He loved to paint portraits. Unfortunately, he lacked the discipline to complete the course and finally lost interest.

I attended Cal–Berkeley, majoring in music and psychology. I tried to convince my parents to let me stay on campus but they refused my request. That's when I moved into the tree house Dad built and made the second floor my bedroom. Its separate entrance through the backyard meant I could come and go at will. It was like having my very own apartment. I furnished it with furniture from the house.

My college years were wonderful. It was the era of Haight Ashbury. I think that's why my parents did not want me to live so far away. I met so many friends and schoolmates who opened my mind to different views of life. I loved to discuss different psychological views with them. For hours, we would have those deep discussions and arguments on life issues. I am sure many of them were stoned, but I never got into the drug scene. Thinking out of the box was cool, though. What an experience.

Only after I graduated from college was I told that Mother Gordon had accumulated a nice sum of money in the bank for me. Talk about a graduation gift! I really didn't have an idea as to what I wanted to do. My best friend was Ola Johnson. We met during our last year in high school. She was African-American and five feet one inch tall. I was five feet eight, but we both were strong willed and competitive.

And we were both well proportioned. We attracted a good share of interested young men and double-dated a lot. For years, we were inseparable, especially after college. Ola's parents moved to San Francisco from Los Angeles. Her dad worked for the IRS and her mother, like mine, was a stay-at-home mom.

Ola and I took drama class together. We also had the same tastes in music and enjoyed each other's company. For our last semester in high school, we were both given parts in the production of the *Sound of Music*. We learned to speak French, which made us very mischievous. Around other people, we would act as if we were visiting from France and did not know how to speak English. People would look at us so strangely. Hearing two young Black women conversing in French was a surprise in itself. It was especially funny when we met boys.

After graduation, Ola decided to go to England to obtain her master's and asked me to come along. I had had enough of college but the idea of going to Europe was so exciting I had to go. With my parents' permission—they let me go only after I promised them I would return to continue my education in September—and after getting my passport and shots, off we went. Yes, a road trip. We found a nice little apartment in England. This was the first time I had ever been out of the country and away from my family. (I encourage every college graduate to take a trip abroad before settling down.) What an experience.

Being in London and Paris and Vienna exposed me to all types of music. I met some of the most extraordinary and talented musicians. However, the most amazing part of Europe to me is the architecture. Buildings and structures that have stood the test of time magnificently and majestically after all these years. I had never seen such beauty. I wanted to see it all. The idea of traveling to places that I read about in school was beyond amazing. What a revelation! While Ola was attending Oxford, I was free to travel on the train to different countries during the week and come back to England on weekends.

There were lots of jazz clubs, art museums, people to meet, and so many things to do. I went everywhere…Germany, Paris, and Rome. Some clubs in England had open-mike night where you could sing with the band. I became a regular. Oh yes, I forgot to mention that I also sang opera. I had taken voice lessons at the S.F. Conservatory of Music. My new life was such a change from life at home. Since I enjoyed singing so much, I decided to make it my career. I didn't drink hard liquor but I learned to love wine.

I was hooked on traveling. I met different people from different cultures and I felt right at home. The ideas we had about life were so different but our respect for each other's philosophy was rich. The experience really expanded my mind. I had men friends of all races. We would take the train or hike the countryside. Since I don't do the camping thing, we would stay in a hostel. It was great! Even though I had promised my parents I would be home in September, it didn't happen. After a few months, Ola and I decided we were staying in Europe forever. I kept telling my parents I would enroll in school, to get my master's, but I didn't. I realized that all those days of practicing the piano, organ, and violin had stored up some very interesting energy. I needed to sow some oats. NO, I was not stupid like "girls gone wild." What is up with that? Why can't girls today take a vacation without baring their breasts, losing their morals, minds, and virginity? Hasn't anyone told them that those pictures will follow them until they die? Anyway, in my day, sowing my oats meant I went to jazz clubs, heard incredible music, and met so many interesting people who just enjoyed life. I even went to Amsterdam.

I visited magnificent cities, ate the best foods, and truly enjoyed my life for the first time. I missed the fall semester and convinced my parents that I would come home before spring semester started. They agreed. Cell phones were not around yet so long distance calls were by operator. We talked long distance, or I would write them a letter.

Needless to say I missed the spring semester and around June of the next year I started to receive calls from my parents proclaiming that if I wasn't home soon, well, let's say money is important to have and if they didn't send it life would have been difficult. I did ask my godmother for some help and, sure enough, she came through. She helped convince my parents to let me stay a little longer. I believe they trusted me even though they weren't happy with my decision. I had not decided what I wanted to do as a career, but I promised them I would be home soon. I went home two months later, in August.

Chapter 10

I returned home confident that I could sing professionally. I'd been independent for over a year so I knew I could make it on my own. It was time to move out of my parents' house. Five weeks and many discussions later, I had convinced my parents. I packed my belongings one Saturday morning and headed for Los Angeles.

Of course, they made me promise to get in contact with Dad's cousin who lived there. I arrived in Los Angeles after a six-hour drive and headed for Cousin Ann's house. As soon as she opened the door, I realized she lived with cats. Immediately, I knew this was not the place for me. When I called home and told my parents about Cousin Ann and that I was getting a place of my own, they agreed. I had more than enough money to survive for several months and make a deposit on an apartment. Mom and Dad knew I was responsible and trusted me but Dad reminded me not to lose my mind. I found a decent hotel and rented a room for a week.

Within three days, I had found a clean furnished apartment and moved in. What a change from living at home. This was a big city. The building had an open courtyard, with a swimming pool in the middle. My apartment was on the second floor, and most of my neighbors were young, in their twenties like me. I felt safe, even though the first night I couldn't sleep listening to all the different sounds and trying to determine if someone was breaking in. After a few nights had passed and nothing happened, my confidence level rose and my fears disappeared. Within three weeks, I had found a job as a secretary in a dentist's office.

Life in Los Angeles was exciting. The city was much bigger than San Francisco and travel time to work was 45 minutes. Since I was not familiar with the long commutes, I was late for my first day at work. My first paycheck was a surprise as well. I was totally shocked when I realized how little money was left after the government took its share. Like my neighbors, I purchased a hibachi, put myself on a budget, and learned to live cheaply. One of my neighbors, Shelly, who I met at the mailbox, told me I needed to find an agent. She encouraged me to get a portfolio with current pictures. Shelly had been in Los Angeles for several years so I took her advice. By the time I gathered all of the required items, three months had passed and I still hadn't sung a note. Many of my neighbors were in the same position as I, people with talent looking to be stars. We shared a lot of information around the pool.

Chapter 11

My first "gig" was for the opening of the Century City Center, in Beverly Hills. Yes, it was a piano bar, not a concert hall, but it was a job. I was as happy as a lark. It was in Beverly Hills, so I was the envy of the apartment complex.

It paid well. I worked from 6:00 to 9:00 p.m. Thursdays to Sundays. It was called the Happy Hour. I didn't sing but I played show tunes. Sometimes I would sneak in a classical song just because.

Carol Anderson had moved in next door to me two weeks after I moved in. We became instant friends. Carol was a dancer from Las Vegas, looking to find a job in a musical or a play. When I told her I got the gig, she asked to see what I was going to wear. According to Carol, I didn't have a clue what to wear and my wardrobe showed it. My clothes were just not appropriate for happy hour. We went shopping. I was not used to having semi-evening wear, so she helped me find some nice dresses. I put myself in her hands and she transformed me from a rabbit into a butterfly. She

48

gave me hairstyling and makeup tips. I bought high heels to match every outfit.

I must say I looked hot. I was 5 feet 8, 38-24-36 and I wore 4-inch stilettos. With my medium dark skin, hazel eyes, black hair, and voluptuous lips (at least that's what I've been told), I walked into a room like I owned it. The first night, I decided to wear a little black dress with the hem just above my knees.

So there I was. I walked in at 5:45 p.m., went to the piano, and took a seat. The bartender, Jack, came over and asked me if I wanted a drink. I told him just water, but put it in a nice glass. He smiled as I started playing. I looked around and realized that I was the only African-American in the place, but that has never been a problem for me.

Once I finished that piece, I received requests for different songs. After a few weeks, I became familiar with the regular customers. Tips were good and I enjoyed flirting. It seems my new wardrobe passed inspection. There were more men than women sitting at the piano, so I was having a blast. My agent, Peter Adams, hadn't come by to see me since he got me the job. We'd talked on the phone and sometimes he would flirt but it really didn't mean anything to me; he was my agent. My boss called Peter and told him how he really was pleased with my work. Peter said he would come by one night to see me. That Friday night he showed up at the hotel while I was playing. I saw him at the door and thought WOW! Peter did a double take because he had not seen me for a few weeks and never in my gig attire. When we would meet in his office, I was in my work clothes. That night I happened to be wearing my little black dress. Since I am so tall, when I play the piano, my piano stool is farther back than most pianists. I need the knee room.

When Peter looked at me, I thought I saw a wow in his eyes too. Yes, it was a wow.

In his office on Wilshire Boulevard, Peter always wore a suit and tie sitting behind his desk. I knew he was tall because when I would come in the room he would stand up. I didn't think of him as a hunk, I saw him as my agent. He talked to me face to face, which is why I liked him. Some of the agents I talked with before choosing him talked only to my chest and I was not impressed. Peter seemed to be genuine and acted as if he wanted to help me. He was polite, not pushy. He sent me to a friend to get the pictures taken for my portfolio. They weren't too expensive so I trusted him.

Peter had the surfer look. Dark blond ponytail hair, blue eyes, and he seemed to be in good shape. I was only interested in getting a job, so I really hadn't paid that much attention to him.

But that Friday night he walked in wearing a dark suit and white shirt unbuttoned. His suit was tailor-made and fit him well. He walked with confidence. As he walked toward me, a strand of blond hair dropped down over one eye. Oh my! I watched how the women in the room perked up. They stared at him like he was a piece of fresh meat. A lady sitting close to the piano asked her friend, "Who's that?" Peter didn't seem to be paying attention to anyone but me. Our eyes met, he smiled, and I smiled back. Have you ever noticed when a man smiles? Some men smile with their eyes, some with their mouth, and some with their body. That night Peter smiled with every part of him and I liked it. His eyes seem to be looking through me. He smiled with just a hint of his teeth showing as he walked toward me.

Suddenly, it seemed as if no one else was there but him. I tried not to stare, so I looked away. I took a deep breath and turned back around. By then, he was standing in front of me at the piano. He was looking down at me, still smiling. I heard him say "Hi." I know I heard him talk to me, but my mouth was dry. My fingers were getting numb. I couldn't remember the song I was playing. What is *wrong* with me, I keep thinking? I was in real trouble. I heard myself say "Hello." Then I felt him gently touch my shoulder. I felt his breath whisper in my ear and I heard him say, "Angie, you look hot." When I was a girl and something really made me laugh, I would just giggle. When his breath hit my ear, I giggled almost uncontrollably—and that had never happened to me before. Peter sat at the piano until I finished the set and asked me out for dinner. I said, "Yes."

We sat at a table near the window; he ordered a bottle of champagne. We talked for hours until I realized it was 2 a.m. It was as if we had just met. He was from Santa Monica and had graduated from UCLA. He was successful because his parents were in the business, and they helped him build his clientele. His family had money. However, he was determined to make it on his own. Peter considered himself a workaholic. He was unmarried and did not have a girlfriend. He said he was not looking for anyone.

Peter walked me to my car and we continued talking. Now it was 3:00 in the morning yet we still had more to say. It was exhausting and exciting. When he came around to open the door, he pulled me to his chest and kissed me lightly on the lips. My knees buckled. Yes! I closed my eyes. Yes, Yes, Yes, I was hooked. After he let me go, I acted as if it had been just a kiss. I smiled, got in the car. He walked away, promising to call me later. I said okay. I needed air. It was a little breezy but if I didn't get any air, I would have exploded. I put the top down and drove home, but I don't remember getting there or undressing. All I remember is sitting on my sofa staring at the wall trying to remember everything that happened to me from the time Peter walked in that door. When I came to myself, it was 9:00 a.m. I called Mother immediately.

Chapter 12

When Mother answered the phone, I just started talking. To her I was rambling, but I needed to get thoughts out of my head. I had never felt like this! I was laughing and smiling, trying to tell her about Peter. She told me to slow down and start from the beginning. What was he like? What kind of job does he have? Who was Peter? When did I meet him? I answered her questions. Finally, she asked me to tell her what happened, and I told her about everything except the kiss. Then she said, "Did you sleep with him"? I shouted, "No, it wasn't like that." I heard a sigh of relief from her. I could hear Daddy in the background asking her "Is anything wrong?" Mom assured him everything was okay. I could hear her smiling. She always had a way of calming me down. I kept talking and she listened without saying a word. Finally, I asked her what was wrong with me. It took her a long time to say anything. She calmly asked me if I liked Peter. Did I like Peter? Wow, I could not answer. The real nerd in me could not answer the question.

Who was I, this silly girl talking a mile a

minute about a man I just kissed for one time? Besides, Peter was my agent. I took a deep breath and said, "Mother you're right. I don't even know this guy." She encouraged me to get to know Peter before making any decisions. I was back to myself. I was breathing again. After we hung up and I took a shower, I poured myself a cup of tea and sat on the balcony thinking. Carol was already outside at the pool. She asked me how was my night so I told her it went well. I did not tell her about Peter; it was nothing.

Since it was Saturday and I had the night off, I stayed home to do chores. Around 2:00 p.m., the phone rang. It was Peter. Before I realized it, I was grinning, and my heart was pounding. He said "Hi Angie," and I was hooked. He said he was thinking about me and had wanted to call earlier. I said "Really?" He told me he did not want to sound too eager. I laughed. We talked until 9:45 p.m. I remember the time because suddenly I realized it was dark in my apartment. For weeks, we would talk on the phone. Peter didn't ask me out, but he would call me every day. I convinced myself we were just friends.

Finally, after three weeks, he asked me out on a date. Getting dressed was the worst experience ever. I could not find the right dress. My hair was not working for me, everything was wrong. When I opened the door, Peter smiled at me. I could not move. Oh no, the feeling was worse this time. Nothing made sense. I wanted him to take me in his arms, but he took my elbow and steered me to his Porsche. I sat and he drove. Neither of us said a word. It was strange but somehow I was comfortable. I really didn't care where we were going, I was just glad to be with him.

We drove a few miles in silence until finally he asked if I was okay. I told him I was okay, and we both started laughing. I think we were both holding our breath. He stopped on the side of the road, pulled me to him, and kissed me. This was not a little kiss. This was a very honest to goodness tongue in my mouth kiss. And I kissed him back. With his face so close to mine he said, "I've wanted to do that for weeks but I was afraid you didn't feel the same way." Oh yes, I felt the same way.

That was the night I became a real woman. I was twenty-three years old. Strange as this may sound, I really just remembered it. My grief dimmed so many good memories that only now are they returning. It has been several years since that happened, and I just realize now that I have been grieving so much I had forgotten about times in my life when I was happy. I feel like I am slowing coming out of a cocoon. I've been hurting for so long that I can't remember when I wasn't hurting.

After several months of steady dating, I moved in with Peter in his house in Beverly Hills. I wanted to get my own band and sing. He found me a pianist, bass guitarist, drummer, and bass player. We were the Five Fingers. Peter got us gigs and parties around town. He enjoyed watching me sing. I would catch him out of the corner of my eye, smiling. I was in love. We both were. He had several other clients, so work was steady, and the money was good, real good.

I stayed home during the day, rehearing, shopping, and just making sure the help was doing their job. It was wonderful but I was feeling so guilty. I didn't tell Mother I was living with Peter but I really think she knew. Each time we talked, she would ask me if I had found a church to attend.

I would always change the subject. This was not how I was raised. I was ashamed, but I was in love. Sometimes we would meet people who had problems with us being a mixed couple, but it did not bother us. I find that if you have money, things are not as difficult to handle. Peter had money. I was getting paid $1500 a night, and was in love. We were happy.

We had been living together for almost six months and I still hadn't visited my parents. I was feeling homesick. I told Peter I was taking the weekend off to drive up to San Francisco. He said he could not get away but that I should go. Even though I had not told Mother I was living with him, I talked about him a lot. I still had the Mustang Dad bought for me. I loved that car.

On Friday, Peter asked me to meet him for lunch. I parked the car. As I was going inside, he met me at the door with this big grin on his face. I asked, "Why are you so happy?" He said, "I have a surprise for you." I turned around. Parked on the street was a brand-new yellow Lamborghini. As I turned to face him, he dangled the keys in front of me. "It's yours." I screamed, "What?" He said that in all the time we had been together, I had never asked him for anything. He was right. I was happy. I had the best life ever. I lived in a Beverly Hills mansion with the man I loved. Now I had a fabulous new car. This was unbelievable. Even if he hadn't bought the car, I knew Peter loved me. He was truly my soul mate.

The next day I drove home to San Francisco to see my parents. Daniel drove me nuts begging me to take him for a ride. Mother, on the other hand, was calm. "It's cute. But why is it yellow?" Dad jumped in, "How much did it cost? How can you afford this?" In the next breath he added, "You know if you get in a wreck, there isn't a lot of car to protect you." Dad believed in big cars. His theory was if you were in a wreck in a big car, you would be protected from serious injuries. All our lives we were protected with Cadillac's. Dad loved driving a black Cadillac. I knew he was proud of me; he was just being Dad. But I felt so guilty.

I could tell Mother was upset, so I asked her to take a ride with me. I drove with the top down to Ocean Beach. We walked on the sand and talked. She asked me if I was happy, and I assured her I was. Mom said she wanted to meet Peter since he sounded so special. She reminded me of my home training and said she was proud that I didn't have a lot of babies running around. She continued to give me the confidence I needed as a woman. She told me not to be a pushover. No matter what happened in life, Mom reminded me, I could always come home. I loved talking to her. She treated me like a grown woman ever though I was her "baby girl." We were having a woman-to-woman talk. She was my best friend. The fact that she respected and was proud of me made me feel good. When we got home, I took Daniel for a ride. I knew he wanted to show off the car to his friends and have them meet his big sister.

After dinner, I gave a mini-concert for my parents. They were so proud and happy. When I woke up the next morning, I could smell those homemade biscuits. Daniel knocked on my bedroom door telling me to get ready so that I would not be late for church. Wow. I really was home. After church, we had Sunday dinner. With hugs and kisses from my family, I left San Francisco, and in five hours, I was home with Peter.

My career was starting to take off. Peter was really promoting us and I was making $3000 for a weekend's work. For parties I made $1000 a night. People liked my voice and I was getting recognition. Peter started encouraging me to record an album. He would tell me he was working on it. I believed him, but I wanted it sooner rather than later. Nine months later, Peter started to change. He worked harder and stayed out later. I suspected there was someone else, but he would always reassure me: I was the only woman. He asked me to marry him a few weeks later, and I said yes. I was ecstatic. I finally told my parents we were living together. They were not happy but accepted the situation, especially after I told Mother we were getting married.

A few months after this, Peter came home so happy I could not understand why. He had some new clients but I did not like them. When I had met Peter, he was confident, hard working, and focused. Now sometimes he missed meetings, seemed a little jumpy, and was even began to take a cavalier attitude toward work. Something was off. We had a dinner party one night and, as usual, I was organizing the house. I was in his office when I found a box on top of his desk. It was an unusual-looking box, but I respected his privacy and had never bothered things in his office.

I opened it and found a white powdery substance. Not knowing what it was, I simply put the box in his top drawer. I made a mental note to tell him where it was the next day. Walking from the kitchen after dinner, Peter grabbed my elbow and pulled me toward his office. He seemed agitated, angry. Not knowing what was going on, I was concerned. He closed the door and asked me if I had seen a box on his desk. I smiled, but he didn't smile back. I told him it was in his desk. He sighed, then opened the drawer, and retrieved the box. I asked, "What's in the box? He would not answer me; instead, he turned around and walked back to the party.

This was shocking, since he had never acted that way before. I followed him. He and the new clients left. He did not come home for hours, but I waited up because I wanted to know what had caused him to act so crazy. I was angry too. I asked, "What are you into?" He assured me it was nothing.

If we were getting married, I told him, there should not be any secrets between us. He smoothed it over. I did not need to be concerned, and nothing had changed between us.

I kept that incident in the back of my mind and starting observing his behavior. His new friends became regulars at our house. They would go to Peter's office, close the door, and lock it, which was quite unusual. Peter had never locked doors. I made myself scarce because I didn't like them. Two weeks later, I came home early from practice to find Peter and his new friends sitting around the pool with this white substance on the table. Then I knew. It was drugs (cocaine) and Peter was very much involved. I will never forget the look on his face when he saw me staring at him.

I ran out of the house, got in my car with him calling my name, asking me not to leave. I couldn't believe it. I was horrified. I wanted to drive home to San Francisco. Instead, I went to a hotel and cried myself to sleep. How could he? Peter was not the same man I fell in love with.

The following day I asked him to meet me at a restaurant because I did not want to go back to his house. His eyes were glazed. He said he had been up all-night and started telling me he really was not into drugs. It was just the "guys" got him to try it. I told him I did not believe him, because he had been acting different for weeks. Finally, he admitted he had been using drugs for two months. I told him this was unacceptable. I would not live with him like this, and I certainly was not going to marry him if he kept acting like a fool. I was mad because he was not honest with me. Besides, I was not going to jail for him or anyone else. I gave him an ultimatum. He promised to stop with the drugs and to get rid of his new clients. This lasted three weeks. Then I found the drugs in the closet and knew it was over. I loved Peter, but I was not going to throw my life in the toilet because he had become a junkie. I was devastated.

I needed time to think. Between crying and packing, I knew I needed to go away. I drove to my parents' house. Mother knew something was wrong when I suddenly showed up. I tried to smile and pretend nothing was wrong, but she knew. Mother always knew when something was wrong. Even when I was a little girl, she could tell just by the look on my face. For weeks, I moped around the house. I never took Peter's calls.

Finally, Mother said she was not going to keep lying to Peter—I needed to talk to him. I told her he and I were not getting married. I never explained why. My parents never pressed me for a reason. Peter called every day. He sent flowers and gifts.

Three weeks later, he was at my door. It was the first time my parents had met him face to face. He looked like the Peter I fell in love with. He was very polite, charming, intelligent, sexy, and very handsome. I sat by Mother while he and Dad talked. I never told them about the drugs, but Dad knew whatever was wrong it was serious. He talked to Peter as if he were my brother, telling him what he expected of him if he was going to marry me. He ended by saying he hoped Peter was a good man. Peter listened to Dad with great respect. I did not believe him. After dinner, we decided to take a walk. He begged and pleaded me to forgive him. I wanted to, I really did, but he had lost my trust and I was deeply hurt. I told him I would think about it. I decided to move home to San Francisco the next week.

The following Monday, I waited until I knew Peter had gone to work. I packed my clothes, put his ring on the desk, and left him a note. I drove the Lamborghini to a used car lot and traded it in for a Lincoln Continental. Later I sent him the money from the sale. I moved back to San Francisco to reclaim my life.

The nightlife really was not me. I was heartbroken and depressed. After crying my eyes out for weeks, I finally decided to get a job. I worked temporary jobs for a while, and then I found this great job as a manager in a law firm. It had good benefits, my co-workers were fun, and I was working to get my life in order. I was first in the office and last to leave, anything to keep my mind off Peter. He called, but I didn't talk to him. He didn't come back up to see me. This went on for two years. I threw myself into my work. I really was a workaholic. I didn't feel like dating. After work, I went home. I still cried myself to sleep. Even though Peter called, I could not convince myself to go back to him. I was growing up.

At twenty-seven years old, I watched all my

friends get married. It seemed like every month I was attending a wedding—I was the wedding singer and getting tired of it. My friends tried to find me a man, but I wasn't interested. On my twenty-eighth birthday, I decided to start dating again. I was still hurt but I was ready. All I needed was the right man in my life, so I started looking.

Life continued. Unexpectedly, Peter called me one-day years later when he was in town. We met for lunch. He looked the same, just a little older. It had turned out for the best that we did not get married. It was not our time. He was a happily married man now with two children. We accepted the fact that what we had was good for a while. My heart still ached but I was not bitter.

Chapter 13

At twenty-nine, what I thought at the time was the most devastating thing that could happen to me, my parents decided to get a divorce. Understand this; I was living in my apartment. My brother was now married and he and his Japanese wife were living in their own place. When Mother and Dad asked us over for dinner and then proclaimed they were getting a divorce, I was shocked and angry. Dad was eighty-eight years old. Mother was sixty-seven. I wondered, "What the hell they were doing? What was strange to me was that there was no anger. They weren't mad, yelling; they were talking to us as if they were planning to go on a vacation. They simply decided to get a divorce. I could not believe what they were saying. Mother said that if we wanted anything we could have it. The house had twenty-one rooms. What did I want? That was far from my mind.

I should have kept the house. After the shock, I got completely crazy. I was mad as hell. Why? Why after almost thirty years of marriage would these old people want to get a divorce? I stormed out of the house vowing never to talk to either one of them again. That lasted two hours. I went back and I listened to them. Both stated that they simply wanted to live by themselves. They still loved each other but they felt they had drifted apart. My question to them was, "What the hell did it matter after thirty years?" I felt they should be able to suffer through the rest of their lives together. However, they made their decision and it was final. After selling the house and the ranch in Santa Rosa, they each got an apartment. I decided it was their money and their house. I could get my own house.

Now that I think about it, my anger was not just at them, it was the fact that this would change my concept of marriage. Selfish, yes! I was also scared for them. I did not know how they would survive not being married, but they did. The future I had imagined for them (and I guess for me) was that—after I got married—I would visit them for Sunday dinners, and they would take care of each other. Well, that's what I always pictured.

Divorce meant they would be apart. Yet my parents had the best divorce ever, if that's possible. First, they got apartments two blocks from each other. Both of their churches built senior apartment buildings. They met for lunch in each other's dining halls and even went to Europe together, twice. Dad took a cruise to Alaska. Mother visited the Holy Land twice, once with Aunt Willie. She and I took two cruises to the Caribbean. They talked on the phone all the time. Who knew this was divorce? I still cannot explain it; all I know is that they were the best of friends until the end of their lives. We still had family meals and took family pictures. Go figure!

Every now and then, I dated, but it never felt right. At thirty-two years old, I had come to the conclusion that marriage was not for me. I remember taking Mother to a wedding and being depressed driving home. Mother asked me what was wrong. I told her I had decided to live alone and not to worry about ever getting married. She laughed at me. She said once I stopped worrying about getting married, the right man would come along. I did not believe that, but sure enough, a few months later I met someone.

I was used to going many places by myself. I was a loner. The young women at my church were just acquaintances. I've always kept my church life and private life separate; I learned that from my parents. Ola was my only close friend. We talked long distance for hours once a week. (After graduation, she had met and married a high school teacher in England. They have two beautiful children and a great house in the countryside near Oxford.) I enjoyed opera and ballet, so I often went by myself. During one performance of *Rigoletto,* I sat next to a tall, charming young man. We talked a while during intermission. His name was Steven Bronnoski. He was cute. When he smiled, his dimples would sink ever so deep in his cheeks. He smiled a lot. Did I mention he was tall? By the time the performance was over, he asked me for my phone number. I actually gave him the right number. I went home and practiced writing my name, Mrs. Angie Bronnoski.

Steven was six feet six, with black hair; brown eyes, wide shoulders, and glasses. He was an attorney with the Alameda County District Attorney's office. Steven was Jewish. He could just smile at me and make me laugh.

Steven and I dated steadily for two

wonderful years. Finally, one night after dinner, he proposed and I accepted. My parents were excited, his not so much. He was busy trying to make a name for himself. I would read about a case in the paper and sometimes he would tell me things without divulging privileged information. I, too, was dedicated to my career. Steven kept me grounded. We realized that to be where we wanted to be, we would have to make sacrifices. We were both still young and did not feel any pressure to get married right away—probably the following year? If we became successful and saved enough money, we would retire when we were fifty-five. Daniel, Mom, and Dad all considered Steven part of the family. He and Dad would talk for hours and even went to baseball games together. We usually had Sunday dinners at Mom's.

When I met his parents, they didn't seem to like me. I tried to attribute it to the fact that they were Jewish and I was Christian, but I knew it was really a racial issue. Steven did not want to admit it and was always trying to convince me it was not because I was African-American. They were not happy with either our relationship or our impending marriage, so we didn't associate with them very much. Steven visited his parents by himself. I learned to live with it, but it did hurt me.

Steven lived in Alameda; I lived in San Francisco. The commute between our apartments wasn't far, just across the bridge. We talked every day for hours even when he or I was traveling. We worked hard during the week but we always went out on weekends. He would forget to call when he was going to be late. I annoyed him while he was reading. I got angry when he forgot my birthday. He would get upset with me whenever I was late for dinner at a restaurant.

I introduced him to crepes. He introduced me to wine festivals and jazz concerts. Many a Sunday we would go sailing on his boat. Since I couldn't swim, I always was strapped into a life jacket, and he would tease me about it. Sometimes, we had brunch in Sausalito or would just go walking in Golden Gate Park. He knew how to calm me down when I was upset. I knew to leave him alone when he was working on a big case. We were good for each other.

Steven's best friend was an attorney he

worked with, Jeff Nickles. Jeff was African-American and a jokester. Whenever Steven called from work, I could always hear Jeff in the background telling him he was whipped and laughing. Jeff was always the life of the party. Brilliant mind, a little loud sometimes, but he had class. Jeff was from New York City and he was dating Monique Laird, a Swedish artist.

When we double dated, we always drew attention. I remember attending the famous San Francisco Black and White Ball. Monique dressed at my place. My gown was white; she wore black. The guys wore black tuxedos and rented a limo. We dined at expensive restaurants. Often we played mind games with strangers because everyone assumed I was with Jeff and Steven was with Monique. The maitre d' would seat Jeff next to me and invite Monique to sit next to Steven. One time the guys immediately got up, changed places, looked at each, turned, and kissed us. Then Jeff proclaimed, "Yes, that be my woman," followed by Steven saying, "Yes, this be my woman too!" Then we all laughed. The maitre d' was embarrassed and apologized. Really, isn't society silly? If you fall in love with someone who treats you right, respects, loves, and cares for you, to hell with anyone else. I have always been comfortable in my skin. Emotionally, I was stronger than Steven. I attributed that to my parents and my home environment.

I was always told I could do anything with perseverance. I know Steven loved me, but he was not strong enough to overcome his family's prejudice. For months and months, I tried to convince him that if he could not stand up to his family, our relationship was in jeopardy. He loved his family very much and I felt our marriage couldn't survive without their acceptance of me. He was in denial. I made it a point to invite his parents for dinner but they always made excuses for not accepting the invitation. Having an interracial marriage was going to be difficult enough for us. His parents' bias was just going to be too stressful. We began to argue about it.

We started drifting apart, making excuses why we could not see each other. I knew if we got married, it would ruin both our lives. I gave him back the ring. We agreed to part ways, but we were both hurt. I think he was somewhat relieved too, even if he did not want to admit it. I wanted him to stand up for us, but he was either unwilling or unable to do so. My parents never had a problem with the race of any men I dated. Their main concern was my happiness. They supported my decision and understood when I told them I was not getting married to Steven. I wanted to get married, but it had to be to the right man.

So again, I thrust myself back in my work and tried to act as if I was completely and utterly happy. Almost a year later, I met Brian McDougal. He was a friend of Ola's husband and was visiting San Francisco. Ola called and asked me to give Brian a tour of the city while he was in town. I agreed. He was from England but his family was originally from Scotland. He was six feet two inches tall, with broad shoulders, black hair, brown eyes, and he spoke with an English/Scottish accent. The first time I heard him call my name was breathtaking. Like Steven, Brian made me laugh a lot. He came to visit for a few weeks but stayed for two years. Within six months, we both were in love. He asked me to marry him.

I talked to his parents over the phone and his

parents talked to my parents. They were eager to meet. This was my Mr. Right. We fit like a glove. He loved me and my parents loved him. His parents loved me and I adored them. All we needed to do was set a date. Have you ever been at that place where everything is right? Your bills are paid, you have the best job ever, money in the bank, stocks are good, you have a man who loves you, and you go to Neiman Marcus to buy a pair of Charles Jourdan shoes for $400 without blinking an eye. That is where I was. Life was great.

Brian and I set a date for the wedding. We really did not want or need a large wedding, so our plans were not extensive. We felt our wedding was between the two of us and we only wanted our immediate families to be present. I only needed Brian. We decided to spend our honeymoon in Tahiti. I lost 10 pounds and was ready to become Mrs. Brian McDougall.

Chapter 14

Longevity is in my family genes. Dad's mother died at one hundred five. Mom's mother died at one hundred one, both of old age. Other relatives have lived until they are in their late eighties or nineties. No one in my family suffers from diabetes, heart ailments, or high blood pressure or any other disease, just old age.

Almost all of my relatives died of "old age"—when you just get real old and forgot to tie your shoes. It was something you expected to happen. Dad's brother, Uncle Andrew, died of cancer, but he smoked and drank for so many years, we knew he would die of something like that. He lived in San Mateo, about 15 miles south of San Francisco, and he was independent until he died. He loved the racetrack and cigars. I remember that whenever he visited our house, he would always give my brother and me money. My Mother's brother Uncle Job, who lived in Mississippi, died of the same disease.

Mom was my rock, my friend, and advisor. I talked to her about everything. When I traveled across the country to sing for conventions or churches, I took her with me. Wherever I gave a concert, she was there. It was always good to know Mother was in the audience. She was my best critic. Looking in her face while I was singing was such a comfort to me. When I needed a friend, Mom was it. I did not have many girlfriends but I had Mom. She would listen to my problems, tell me what I needed to hear and advise me when I needed advice. I knew whatever we talked about was always, always between her and me. Mother would comfort me when I was depressed. Dad would talk to me and impart his words of wisdom about men and money matters. With Mom, I could talk frankly about people and relationships. That mature relationship mothers and daughters have is special. When I was a child, she allowed me to spread my wings but was always there to pick me up when I lost my way.

As a woman, she respected my decisions and discussed them with me, but ultimately she let me make the choice. There were times when we strongly disagreed but most of the time she would be right.

Mother was a lady. Even in her seventies, she still sewed, knitted, and kept herself well dressed. She walked and talked with dignity. She was active in many of the senior activities in her building. If there was a fashion show, Mother was always asked to participate. She would design an outfit and model it. Everyone in the building knew and respected her. Some of the senior men would ask her for a date, but she would just laugh and walk away.

My parents still had lunch together almost every week. She would visit his senior complex, which was two blocks away, or he would visit hers. She lived across the street from her church. She volunteered to play the piano for the B.T.U., better known as the Baptist Training Union. Of course, some of the women did not like her because she didn't gossip or feel the need to socialize with them during the week. That was their problem. She was a loner. Besides, she was always busy writing in her book or sewing something. Mom attended the church prayer meetings on Wednesday nights and street witnessing on Saturdays.

Mother is the only lady I know who in her

seventies drove a two-door Pontiac Firebird convertible with the top down and enjoyed it. I mean she *drove* that car. It was burgundy with a black convertible top. When Mom was coming to my apartment, all I had to do was to look out the window and there she was with the top down, driving fast. I loved it. I still smile when I think of her and how she looked in that car. Many a day other drivers on the road would stare at us, as this elderly lady would pass them on the freeway driving 70 mph. She loved life and lived it well. Grass did not grow underneath her feet. Often I would call and not get an answer. I knew she was out either doing something to keep active at the church or participating in some senior activity.

Dad was the same way. Every morning he would take his constitutional walk of two miles or more. He was always busy doing something, at his church or helping a fellow church member. Even after they divorced, they remained active in their churches. Dad was a well-respected deacon for over fifty years at the same church. Everyone in the community loved and respected him. His weakness was mud baths. He loved having mud baths so much that every other weekend he would drive up north over 100 miles to Calistoga, to get a mud bath. His skin was smooth and clear. I think that is why he looked so young. Years later, I discovered that he was not going alone. He kept his private life private. WOW!

Chapter 15

The first time I noticed Mother was in difficulty was on a Saturday night. Mother had received a call from Nathaniel, my first cousin, to tell us that his mother, Mom's sister, had suffered an aneurysm of the brain. She was in a coma. He asked Mother to come to St. Louis as soon as possible. She and Aunt Willie were very close. They were much closer than any of her other brothers and sisters. Mother was the youngest girl and Aunt Willie was born a year before her. They talked on the phone every week. Aunt Willie was still managing my grandparents' farm in Mississippi and sent us pecans and peaches every September. Mother made preserves and pecan pies all winter long.

This was bad. It was very bad. Until that day, the word *aneurysm* never meant anything to me. I cannot remember ever hearing the word, especially in the context of illness in our family. I called Brian. He came right over and we scheduled a flight to St. Louis that night. He wanted to go with me, but I convinced him I could handle the situation. I packed and he drove me to Mother's place. With the help of Daniel, Mother was packed and ready to go. During the flight, she was very quiet. I really didn't have much to say, especially because I wasn't sure what to expect when we arrived in St. Louis. I was nervous and sad for Mother. Upon landing, I rented a car and we drove directly to the hospital. I called my secretary and left a voice mail explaining what had happened. I told her to cancel my appointments indefinitely.

When we arrived at the hospital, I spoke with the doctors. The doctors indicated Aunt Willie was brain-dead and they did not expect her to live. A neighbor had found her on the floor in her home. She had been unconscious for several hours. If you are unaccustomed to sickness or illness, then you can imagine what a traumatic experience this was for my uncle, cousin, Mother, and me, most especially Mother.

Aunt Willie was Mother's big sister, the last living sibling she had. They went to the Holy Land twice, and on two cruises. Whenever we visited Aunt Willie, Mom would turn into a little sister. Mother enjoyed it. They would laugh for hours telling stories of things that happened to them while growing up.

Mother would always talk about how she and Aunt Willie were on the woman's basketball team in college. She said Aunt Willie was the best player on the team. Aunt Willie would always tell us how my grandparents were so proud when Mother was chosen as the valedictorian of her class. Her theme was "Through difficulties we conquer." Aunt Willie said Granddad Levi, my grandfather, and Della, my grandmother, packed all her sisters and brothers in a wagon to attend graduation. I knew Mother had skills.

After waiting in the hospital for several hours, we drove to my aunt's house to get some rest. I found a dictionary and looked up the word. *Aneurysm.* Yes, the doctors explained that a blood vessel burst in Aunt Willie's head. She was being kept alive with the help of a breathing machine. I was in shock, so I could not imagine what Mother was feeling. That scared me. I prayed for a miracle and asked God to let my aunt recover.

Aunt Willie was eighty-eight years old but she was a strong and healthy woman. She had no physical or mental problems and was always on the move. She owned nine homes and two apartment buildings. She created a Feed the Homeless organization for her church—setting up food pickups from grocery and department stores. She managed the church halfway house for men. Aunt Willie ran them all, with very little help from my uncle. He was frail and not too ambitious. He had not worked for years and sometimes he drank too much. I was oblivious to anything more than a headache, so I was in denial.

When I spoke with Brian, I explained the situation. He tried to tell me that even if she recovered, she would never be the same. He wanted to join me, but I convinced him that I could handle it, and that I was all right. What I realize now is that I went through this whole experience in shock, yet I could still function. The automatic pilot in my brain took over to process data so that I appeared to be functioning well.

My cousin Nathaniel was taking this hard. He was in no condition to make real decisions. Nathaniel was thirty-two years old, an only child, and inconsolable. I had to take charge. Aunt

Willie's attorney called and asked if I would come by his office. This shocked me because I did not know anyone in St. Louis except my aunt. How did Nathaniel know me? Who was this guy? All these questions ran through my head. He had contacted the doctor and was given the status of her condition.

Before going back to the hospital, I went to Nathaniel's office. He apologized and was sorry to meet me under these circumstances. He told me I needed to be aware that Aunt Willie had made me the executor of her estate, including power of attorney of her medical affairs. He told me that in her will, if ever she was incapacitated and unable to make decisions, I was in charge. He further indicated that she did not want to remain alive on life support. I was to make sure that her wishes were kept. I was to remain the executor of her estate for one year. I had the power of attorney to have her removed from the breathing machine. What! Was he kidding me? I started crying. I sat listening to this man tell me that I now had my aunt's life in my hands. Oh my God. Apparently, Nathaniel was aware of her decision. I met Mother and Nathaniel at the hospital. I did not talk about meeting my cousin because I was confused and scared. We stayed for several hours then went home. When Brian and I talked that evening, I never mentioned the meeting.

The next day we went back to continue our vigil but there was no change in her condition. The doctor asked if I was ready to make a decision, but I was not. After praying and discussing this with Mom and my cousin, we decided to wait to see if she would improve before making a final decision. Unless you have ever been in my position, you have no idea what it means to have that responsibility. This was a living person. She was a mother, a wife, who was now in a condition where I had to decide if she lived or died. This was unnatural. I felt as if I was having an out-of-body experience. I heard, I reacted, but my mind could not grasp the finality of the situation.

Whatever her medical status, this was my aunt, a part of me, God forbid. To have to live with that image, that burden, that question as to whether I was doing the right thing, I did not feel I could live with it. For those who have had to make that decision, I pray for you. To live with that decision was beyond my comprehension.

Two days later, there was no change; she was indeed brain-dead. We prayed at my aunt's bedside. I prayed that God would help me. Reluctantly, I made the decision to pull the plug the next day. However, early that morning we received a call from the hospital telling us Aunt Willie had passed away during the night. If the doctors had carried out that decision of mine, I do not know how I would be today.

We immediately went to the hospital because Mother wanted to see her sister. She cried, looked at me, and said, "I'm the last one." I knew what she meant. She indeed was the last of fourteen children. My stomach knotted up. I felt like screaming and yelling. Instead, I looked at her and told her she would always have me to take care of her. She was not going to be alone. I promised her she would never be alone.

As we went through the funeral process, Mother appeared to be taking it well. Occasionally I would hear her crying, when she was alone, but she was a strong person. Aunt Willie had prepaid for everything. She even had the burial dress marked in her closet. I made sure everything went the way she wanted it to. We were never hungry because the neighbors constantly brought food for us. My uncle took it the hardest. We reminded him that God knows best, but I think he regretted the way he had treated my aunt.

Being their only child, Nathaniel was a wreck, but his girlfriend supported him and helped comfort him. Several days after the funeral, we were all asked to meet with the attorney. He read the will. My aunt left Nathaniel six houses and an apartment building along with $30,000 in cash. She gave my mother an apartment building and me a house. My uncle was to remain in the house he lived in.

There were no mortgages on any of the properties. All we had to do was to collect the rents, maintain the properties, and pay the taxes and insurance, beginning the following year. I was to manage the homes and apartments for one year. Collect rents, pay bills, utilities, etc. My cousin was to live in one of the houses and maintain it for a year. It was clear why she made me the executor of her estate. I was the oldest and I think Aunt Willie felt Nathaniel needed time to really understand the value of assets. Mother had no complaints.

We stayed an extra week so I could get things in order with the attorney. Brian called me every day. He was my rock. Many times, I would call him and cry on his shoulder. He comforted me. I convinced him not to come across country. Mother loved talking with Brian. He sent her flowers, which pleased her. After talking to him, she would smile and tell me how blessed I was to have him in my life. I agreed. He was the best. Dad called a few times and sent flowers, which really cheered Mom. Daniel called every day. He and Nathaniel would talk for hours. When we were young, when we visited my aunt for summer vacations, Daniel and Nathaniel were inseparable. They would go fishing or bike riding for hours alone. They were so much alike. Nathaniel taught Daniel how to catch fireflies (there are no fireflies in San Francisco). We were all coping as best we could.

Now that I think about it, I completely ignored a warning sign about Mother's difficulty. That Sunday night we left the hospital and stayed at my aunt's house. Mother cooked dinner and we all went to bed. My mother was in my aunt's bedroom. I took the guest bedroom. Around 3:00 in the morning, I found Mother walking in the dark, in the hallway. She was startled when I turned on the light. She looked at me and asked, "Where are we?" I explained to her the events of the day and walked her back to the bedroom. I tucked her in and told her to go back to sleep. I remember this vividly. I attributed the confusion to shock. This scared me. Suddenly, I saw my mother as a scared child. I had never seen her so vulnerable and fragile. Heck, she was the backbone of the family. I shrugged those feelings off. Sure, she was just in shock. The following morning Mother was back to herself. There was no other evidence of change for several months.

Mothers' first priority when we got back to San Francisco was to make sure her own funeral arrangements were updated. She became somewhat obsessed with making sure Daniel and I knew where all her important papers were located. She visited the funeral home and spoke with the director. She made sure the plots; headstones, caskets, and even our own funeral programs were all in order (she had bought burial plots for all of us when we were fifteen years old). Now she was making sure there would be no problems if anything happened to her. She rewrote her will. I realized then that my aunt's death had really affected her, but she appeared to be handling the situation well. Brian and I talked about it. He convinced me it was expected and I agreed. We decided to wait a few months before making the final plans for our marriage. I still didn't notice any other changes in Mother's behavior. I worked. I called her every day and visited with her twice a week. Daniel and I continued our separate routines. It was working.

A few months later, I received a call at work that Daniel was in the hospital. I rushed to the emergency room. I found him hooked up to monitors and machines. He was unconscious. I had never seen my brother so sick. The doctor told me he had suffered kidney failure and needed a kidney transplant. The doctor said Daniel had high blood pressure, which resulted in renal failure. Until they found a kidney, he would need dialysis.

I offered my kidney, but I was not a match. Daniel's name was added to the national database of patients who need transplants. In order to have dialysis, he needed to have a shunt placed in a vein in his arm, which required surgery. I was scared. None of us had ever needed surgery.

I called Brian. He brought my parents to the hospital. When Daniel regained consciousness, we all talked about the situation. My parents seemed calm but were extremely concerned. Dad as always was quiet, but I knew he was upset. Brian was my support. This was our first real family crisis. I knew Daniel was as scared as I was. He agreed to have the surgery for the shunt. Like me, he was in shock and could not understand why this had happened to him. We were all so unprepared for this. Brian was supportive and caring.

I called my boss and requested a week off from work. The surgery was scheduled for the next day. After I left the hospital, I went to Mother's, packed a suitcase, and brought her to my house. It was clear that I was going to have to take care of Daniel and Mother. Well into his nineties, Dad was not able to help me.

The surgery was a success. Daniel would be released within two days to stay with Mother during his recovery. Sometimes Mother didn't seem to understand why Daniel was in the hospital, but I would explain it to her. She enjoyed living with me, and I enjoyed having her. And one night, Brian came over and cooked dinner for us. He was busy at work but we talked for hours every day.

Like most men, Daniel never went to the doctor until something major was bothering him. Years earlier, he had married his Japanese sweetheart. That lasted for three years. For the last year or so, he had been staying alone. According to the doctor, he had been drinking a lot, which contributed to the high blood pressure. He worked for the city parks and recreation as a gardener. After the surgery, he filed for disability because he was unable to work. He was having a hard time with the dialysis. Sometimes he would be so tired he could hardly stay awake. I was glad when Mother insisted he move in with her. I knew they could help each other. He needed dialysis three times a week, and she enjoyed taking care of him. It made her feel needed, and it was good for both of them. I was relieved I didn't have to take care of them. Brian and I continued making plans for our wedding and the move to New York. I was really looking forward to our new life together.

When Mother and I were together, I didn't notice any major changes in her behavior. Daniel hadn't noticed any real changes either. He said Mother didn't cook as much as she used to. Brian and I visited her at least once a week. She still talked about her funeral arrangements, but I attributed that to the fact that she was still grieving from the loss of her sister. We were slowly getting back to our normal routines.

One day while I was visiting Mother, a neighbor stopped by to tell me Mother had gotten lost while driving to the supermarket. Safeway is only four blocks from her apartment. When I asked Mom about it, she denied it ever happened. At the time, I shrugged it off. On another occasion, I visited her and she asked me, "What day is it?" I told her, but in twenty minutes, she repeated the question. Before I left, she asked me again. I called Daniel and asked him if he had observed any changes in Mom. He said that sometimes she would forget little things but nothing major. I decided to spend some time with her myself.

Mother had never had any physical problems. I would make two medical appointments for her a year. One exam was for a complete physical. The other was for her vision. Those were the only medical appointments she had ever needed. Brian had to go on a business trip. It was a good time to have her spend some time with me.

On Friday night, I picked her up and brought her to my place. When we arrived, she asked me several times, "Where are we?" I told her that she was at my place and she smiled. Later she asked me the same question. We had dinner, watched a movie, and went to bed. She couldn't remember where the bathroom was located. I left the night-light on to help her in case she had to get up during the night. Mother was getting old so I attributed the confusion to "old age." I did not observe any other incidents that week, so I concluded she was all right. Daniel and I decided to stay close to her. Brian offered to call and talk to her every day. We postponed the wedding for a few months. Daniel agreed to continue to stay with her, even though he was looking for a place of his own. I talked to her several times a day. I was starting to get concerned.

Mom was still driving her Pontiac Firebird 350. She loved that car. She was still very independent. She still cooked some marvelous meals. She participated in fashion shows and sewing classes that were offered in her building. Mother had always believed in clean dishes, made up beds, and everything in its place. During one of my visits, I noticed she had a pile of clothes on a chair in her bedroom. I asked her why were they there. Mother said she was spring-cleaning, which sounded reasonable to me. Mother always had spring and fall cleanings. I don't know if it is a Black thing, but that is what we did in our house. In September, we rearranged all the clothes in our closets. Summer clothes were placed in the back of the closet or discarded if they were old. Winter clothes were moved to the front of the closet for easy access. There was never any clutter in her house. Mother always changed her closets from summer clothes to the winter, including shoes and linen.

I decided to help, so I took the winter clothes out and put the summer clothes away. However, when I came back to her place a few days later the summer clothes were back on the chair. Again, I asked her why. She said she was putting them away because they were summer clothes. I explained to her that we'd put the summer clothes away already. I put the winter clothes in the back of the closet. Then I noticed she had dirty and clean clothes in the same drawer. Mother would never do that. I asked her, "When was the last time she'd taken a bath?" She said that morning. There weren't any wet towels in the hamper. When I asked her again, she changed her story and told me it was "last night."

When Daniel came home, I asked him what he had observed Mother doing that was different. He said she had not taken a bath for several days. I filled the tub with water and insisted she take a bath. She adamantly denied that she needed a bath but took one anyway. I knew that was one of the symptoms of dementia but it hurt me to have to ask her. When we finished, she proclaimed that she felt good. While she was in the tub, I went through her drawers and found all kinds of soiled clothes placed back in the drawer with the clean clothes. I gathered her dirty clothes and took them to my house to launder. From then on, I knew that I needed to do her laundry. I was embarrassed for her. I asked, "How are you feeling?" She insisted she was fine. I asked her, "When was the last time you cooked?" That morning, she said. Daniel told me Mom had not cooked anything for quite some time. He was cooking. She again asked me, "What day is it?" I told her.

Brian arrived, I cooked, and we all played Scrabble as usual. Around 8:30, she appeared to be tired, so I put her to bed. Mother loved Brian and treated him like her son. Daniel and Brian got along like brothers, teasing each other as men do. Daniel stayed with her, so Brian and I left. We bought a bottle of wine and went to my place for the evening. Now I was starting to worry. What would happen when I moved to New York? I had to think about the future. I never told Brian what had happened before he arrived at Mom's—that was a private matter. I did not want him to know how scared I was, so I pretended everything was all right. This was my problem, my family. Mother might have some kind of mental problem, but I didn't want to jump to the wrong conclusion. We decided to finalize our wedding plans and to marry later in January. I was excited and scared. I had to find out what was happening with Mother and yet I was afraid to know.

Something was wrong. Something was very wrong. Daniel and I decided to make an appointment with a facility that specialized in treating seniors for mental and physical conditions. I was optimistic. If she needed medication, we would make sure she took the medication. We had a plan and convinced ourselves we could handle the problem.

Chapter 16

On the day of the exam, I called Mother and told her I would pick her up in twenty minutes. When I arrived at her place, she wasn't dressed. She asked, "Why didn't you tell me you were coming?" I told her I just called, but she insisted she did not know I was coming. I got her dressed and we left for the doctor's office. While in the waiting room, she kept asking why we were there. I told her she was getting her yearly checkup. Later she asked again. I gave the same response. She accepted that explanation and stopped asking me. During the examination, she told the doctor there was nothing wrong. After the physical exam, he agreed. He said for her age (79), she was in excellent condition. When the doctor asked me about her health, I told him that she had no physical ailments. The only time Mother had to go to the hospital was when she had broken her little toe. She only went because Dad insisted she go.

That had been at least twenty-five years earlier. For their anniversary, Dad purchased a very expensive bedroom set with a canopy, which she loved. One day while she was cleaning, she struck her little toe against the leg of the bed. Her toe looked very bruised and swollen, but Mother prepared a home remedy and kept on going. Being from the South, my parents knew all kinds of treatment for different ailments. After a week and a half, she was still hobbling around the house. Dad insisted she have it checked out. We got in the car and he drove to the hospital.

How shocked the doctor was when he found out she had been walking on that foot for over a week. She had even worn her high heels to church the previous Sunday. The doctor told her she had a broken toe and immediately put her in a cast, which went up to her knee. Having to wear a cast on didn't set well with her, she was not happy. And talk about disbelief—we were shocked when we saw her walking down the hall on crutches, with her leg in a cast.

She received a follow-up appointment in six weeks, and that cast was supposed to stay on the whole time. Mother decided after four and a half weeks she was not only annoyed with the inconvenience of having to wear a cast, she didn't liked how it looked on her. She proclaimed she was healed and cut it off all by her. That cast never had a chance against her hammer and chisel. I came home from school and the poor thing was standing up in the living room, by itself. I remember asking her what the doctor said. She walked past me and said, "About what?" I asked her what the doctor had said about the condition of her toe. She looked at me and smiled, "I guess he would say I'm healed because I feel fine." She laughed and I could not help but laugh with her. Dad came home, looked at the cast, and in his unemotional manner turned to her and said, "Oh you couldn't wait." He smiled, shook his head, and walked away. That was the only time she ever had what could be considered a serious problem. She never limped and wore high heels the next Sunday. Mother was very healthy.

Now another doctor was talking to her. He asked, "What day is it?" She gave the wrong answer. I was perplexed. I began to answer the questions for her. Of course, my answers were different from hers. He asked questions like, "What day is it? What year? Who is the president of the USA? She passed the physical examination with no problems, but she failed the mental questions. I explained to the doctor what I had observed over the last few weeks. He said she needed more tests. Reluctantly I agreed. We made an appointment for the next week.

I took Mother to the appointment. Two physicians conducted the tests. One physician again examined Mother physically, and the other had her perform some psychological tests. At the conclusion of the examination, I was asked to wait outside until the doctors consulted with each other.

After a while, Mother and I were escorted into the conference room. The doctors sat at one end of the table, Mother and I were at the other end. They told me Mother was in perfect health. However, they also told me she had the beginning signs of Alzheimer's.

Where were you when you first heard the word *Alzheimer*? I know exactly where I was. Each doctor facing me had a report. Their looks said; I wish I could help. My stomach instantly developed a knot, my heartbeat slowed, and my mind raced. What was Alzheimer's? Is it some kind of stroke, brain tumor, or what? I heard them say words like dementia, no cure, and deterioration of the brain. I heard those words but they were not registering. If she was healthy physically, then this cannot be so bad. I was going to get a second opinion.

They gave me brochures, they told me about dementia, but I was in shock. Just tell me Mother has old age; that is what I expected to hear.

As I drove home, so many things were going through my mind. Medication, had I asked about medication? Then I remembered, the doctors said there was no medication for this. What else had I forgotten to ask? My brain was spinning. I called Daniel and told him to meet me at Mother's place. I called Brian and told him everything is okay. Mother is healthy as always. I lied. I lied. I cannot believe I lied. I could not tell him. All I could think about was that word Alzheimer's. They had to be wrong. This was old age. I was getting married and moving to New York in a few months. This *had to be* old age!

What the hell was Alzheimer's? Where did it come from? What is dementia? What is that? I was mad. Mad at what the doctors told me—Mother was no longer perfect. She couldn't take care of herself anymore. And I was mad, mad at whatever was happening to her, to my best friend. She is my support when all else fails. THIS IS MY MOTHER. Alzheimer has changed my life forever. I don't mean to sound selfish, because it certainly affected Mother's life worse than mine. But the expectations for my life changed dramatically and forever.

What could I blame for this condition? Was it something she ate? What caused this mess? How can we get it fixed? I took Mother back to her place. I was angry, but at the time, I did not understand why. I subconsciously realized I was going to have to take care of my mother. No question, I would have to take care of my mother. And I had no idea what form that care would take.

All my life, words like Alzheimer's, dementia, caregiver, and anything associated with taking care of my parents never, ever entered my mind. Everyone believes that our parents will grow old, live independently, be able to take care of each other, and not need help or assistance from their children. That is exactly what I expected. I needed that to happen, especially now.

In the Black community, Alzheimer's was a

foreign word and meant nothing to me. In fact, my first questions to the physicians were, "What type of medication would she have to take to resolve this problem?" They looked at me with astonishment and explained that there was no cure. They emphasized that this condition would get worse. The final stage would be dementia and death. More words I did not want to hear.

Cancer, renal failure, heart disease are serious diseases, not Alzheimer. I looked at my healthy little mother and I was in disbelief. No, I would not accept this. Obviously, these people have misdiagnosed her condition. All we are dealing with is old age. That is what I said and that is how I felt. I would not, could not in any way believe that Mother—who had never been sick a day in her life—was suffering from something unseen and certainly unknown to me. According to them, there was no cure. No! No! This was my mother.

Mother is physically well, healthy—she doesn't look any less intelligent, not at all. Old age, that is all the hell this is. They gave me the results of the test and I did not read it. As far as I was concerned, it was old age. They just misdiagnosed her; doctors do that. So I told my brother and, like me, he wouldn't believe them. I took my mother home.

Chapter 17

Unrealistic as it sounds, we set our minds on the premise that Mother was suffering from old age and kept that belief for almost a year. No, I was not taking her to another doctor. We developed a plan. We treated her ourselves. We just knew we could make her remember things. We began a routine. Daniel stayed with Mother and I went by the house more often to help. That was the plan. Occasionally, Brian and I would have dinner. We tried to make time for us. With both of us working, me trying to maintain two households, and making plans for a wedding, I was stretched very thin. Even though I loved Brian with all my heart, I tried not to impose my emotional distress on him. Perhaps it was because my parents raised us to be very private. Many a time I would tell Brian I was handling the situation well, but it really had a big effect on our relationship. Both physical and mentally I was losing me.

I was reactive. If a problem arose, I reacted. I noticed that my focus on getting married was starting to waver. Many a day, I would sit alone trying to determine if it was fair for me to entangle Brian in this situation. I didn't feel it was, even though he reassured me he was with me all the way. I turned the question over and over. I started feeling anger and resentment—anger because I was in this situation and resentment that I could not walk away from it. Brian and I started arguing about the most trivial things. I was not as open with him, and he got more and angry with me. My lack of interest in him convinced him I didn't love him, which just wasn't true. Absorbed in adjusting to my life with Mother, I was protecting him from me.

On the anniversary of my aunt's death, I flew back to St. Louis to meet with the attorney. I needed to finalize my executor's duties and turn the properties and responsibilities over to my cousin Nathaniel. Occasionally, he and I had talked. And his conversations with Brian helped him mature. By the time the year ended, Nathaniel knew what a blessing he had. No one outside of our family knew our business. I found a property manager to manage my properties and flew home.

I was still in denial but I did know something was wrong, something was very wrong with Mother. So what did I do? I finally found books and pamphlets and begin to read literature about Alzheimer's. The more I read, the more I worried that the test could be right. No. I refused to believe it. How could this be happening to Mother? No one on her side of the family ever had this condition. Dad's family never had it. Dad was ninety-seven and he could remember everything. No, it was just old age. That is what I kept telling myself.

Multi-tasking took on a completely new meaning for me. As a corporate manager, I worked sometimes ten hours a day. I loved my job. I was good at it, so good that I got a promotion and needed to travel more. I kept my private life and my work life separate. I kept them separate because I acted like two different people. At work, I appeared all put together, cheerful and focused on my job. With more traveling, came more stress. Now I had to balance traveling with working around Daniel's dialysis schedule. And he kept a close eye on Mother to make sure she was safe. I managed her finances and visited her at least three times a week to give her baths. We took turns doing the laundry. I provided Daniel money to take care of the household expenses. All this while trying to spend quality time with Brian, to plan our wedding, to continue to be the minister of music at my church, and to act as if everything was just peachy.

No one knew about the other side of me. The ME who arrived home immediately turned on the TV, took a shower or bath, got in bed, curled up in a fetal position, and cried every night. Sometimes I would cry so long that when I stopped, it was time to get up and go to work. I cried because my life was all messed up. I was lying to a man who loved me with all his heart. I did not want Brian to pity me; he deserved better. He deserved love, happiness, and a great life. I wanted to be happy. My mother deserved to live a life of happiness but I was losing her mentally. I was losing everything. Everything that I had wanted, expected, and needed was starting to disintegrate, and I did not know how to stop it.

Often, I would call Dad and talk to him. He listened to me and tried to give me advice. Dad told me to change what I could, and not worry about the things I could not. That is hard to do.

Brian was becoming increasingly irritated with me. I still could not bring myself to tell him I was a phony. I was *not* okay. I was scared. How could I move to New York or get married, knowing Mother could not take care of herself without me? Daniel was helpful, but he was a man and there were certain things he could not and should not have to do. I needed to make sure Mother took a bath. I needed to wash her clothes. Yes, I still found soiled clothes in the dresser drawer, but I would come by, take the dirty laundry, and give her a bath.

I knew Daniel needed space, so on weekends I would bring Mom to my house. We would do girl things. I would take her to the nail shop for a manicure and pedicure. When we got home, I would give her a bath and do her hair. We watched TV and talked for hours. I tried to encourage her to help plan the wedding. I wanted to make her mentally alert. Stimulate her memory. We played Scrabble a lot. I forced her to read the *TV Guide* to help her make decisions. And she always read the Bible. I would make up some kind of problem and ask her advice to stimulate her analysis on how to resolve the problem.

Brian visited Mother often. He would take her for dinner or a movie. As the weeks and months passed, I started to see her change. I also started to see Brian change. Initially I know he was willing to help, but as time passed, I could see he was uncomfortable. Mother would ask me, "What should I wear"? She was starting to depend on Daniel and me to make all her decisions.

I knew I could not devote as much time to Brian as I wanted. And then I began to envision me with Alzheimer. He would have to take care of me, and I could not let that happen. I did not want to picture Brian having to bathe me, or me not knowing who he was. I could not and would not let that happen to Brian, I loved him too much. In November, I made the decision. It was during Thanksgiving dinner when I really knew I could not get married. Mother did not cook anymore, so I was planning dinner at my house.

I took off work Wednesday and purchased all the ingredients for the next day's meal. Daniel drove Mother to my house after work that afternoon. I cooked a peach cobbler and a 7-up cake, which I knew were Mom's favorites. She wanted to help so I encouraged her to sit and tell me what ingredients I needed. I was always trying to stimulate her mind and have her feel like she was helping. Daniel watched football. Dad had already made plans, so he wouldn't be coming to dinner. I cooked turkey, Cornish hens, macaroni and cheese, peas, carrots; made dressing and dinner rolls. We would also have cranberry sauce and eggnog. After work, Brian had come over with wine to help me finish cooking. We were in the kitchen laughing, grinning, and acting foolish. Suddenly Mother came in and asked me, "Where is the bathroom?" I told her. Brian and I went on cooking but I remember the look on his face. He ordered pizza since we were saving dinner for the next day. Later we all played Scrabble.

Brian and I took a walk late that evening. I stopped, grabbed him, and asked him to hold me in his arms. He was stunned and asked what was wrong. Nothing was wrong, I said. I just needed him to hold me in his arms and make the world go away. We stood there for almost twenty minutes. I was trying to remember what his hugs felt like. Oh God, I didn't want to let him go. We kissed and I watched him drive away.

I realized that I was shaking. I sat on the steps numb. It was as if I was having an out-of-body experience. I was watching Brian, the man I loved with all my heart, and who loved me. Then I was looking at what was happening to me. Yes, I was trapped. I felt like I was in a cocoon and it was closing in around me and I could not get out. I *had* to be in it. I really did not want to drag Brian into it. He deserved better. I knew the answer. Only I could make a decision.

My decision would impact the rest of our lives. It has been a long time since that day but I never told anyone. Not until now. I said I would die before revealing that decision. I wanted to save him. Do I regret it? No. What I regret is not sharing my feelings with Brian and allowing him the opportunity to make a decision with me. I didn't trust him enough. My decision was selfish. To this day, I do not know if Brian would have stayed, but at the time, I felt I was right.

As I was growing up, Mother and I would have discussions, and I would express my concerns about life. My argument was that I was getting old.

For years, I would ask her, "Do you think I'll ever get married?" and she would tell me yes. Mother would say, "You'll find the man who will make you happy." And I found the right man who made me happy but I gave him up. Maybe I was a coward. I do not know; perhaps I will never know.

When I walked back into the house and looked at Daniel and Mother, I knew I had to accept the fact that this was my cocoon. There could be no one else in it but the three of us. It would be unfair to ask the man I love to share this experience. No one else should bear the burden. I would not allow that to happen to him. Brian was my life. Brian was my love. Brian was my happiness but I had to let him go. It's strange how our minds work, because I remember that day only now. I am speechless. It's incredible how our minds can take a devastating situation and bury it so deep in our subconscious. I knew what I had to do.

Brian came for breakfast the next day and the four of us spent the day together. I had Mother help me finish dinner while Brian and Daniel watched football. I remember standing in the doorway looking at them and thinking how blessed

I was. I was also crying inside. I was giving up my life for my mother. I hated this. After dinner, we played Scrabble and had the best Thanksgiving I would ever have again. Brian talked about what life was going to be like next year in our own house. Brian wanted Mother to stay with us; he knew she couldn't live alone.

Brian wanted children. I wanted children. He laughed at the thought of how they would look or how they would act. He said that with my stubborn streak and his passion and calmness our kids would be either hyperactive or nerds, but no matter, they would be our beautiful children. I looked into his eyes and started to cry. He asked me what was wrong; I told him how happy he made me feel. He wiped my eyes and kissed me softly on the lips. All he said was, "I'm glad, because I love you with all my heart." Brian never knew what I was really crying about. I had made up my mind, and I knew I would break his heart. My heart was already broken for what I knew I was giving up. That was the last Thanksgiving when I was really, really, happy.

I had to focus on Mother. Brian called me

several times that next week but I would not return his calls. He called Daniel and asked if everything was okay. Daniel asked me several times why I was acting so crazy, and why wouldn't I call Brian. I blamed it on work or church. I promised Daniel I would call Brian, but I did not. The next weekend Brian came by my place but I didn't answer the door. He called and left messages.

Finally, I called him and set up a date the next night so we could talk. I tried to act normal and cooked dinner. There was a strange silence between us, which we had never had before. I knew he was frustrated, angry, and confused, with good reason. He asked me why I was acting so different. I took a deep breath. I had played this discussion in my head for the past week. I did not want it to sound like I had lost my mind. I did not want to hurt him, but hurt him I would.

I explained the concerns I had over Mother's health. I did not want to go into detail, but I needed him to see my side of the story. The lump in my throat hurt. I sat across from him because I could not bear to be near him. I really wanted him to hold me in his arms. I needed to cry on his shoulders. I knew I needed that, but I held back. I loved him so much it hurt. As much as I loved him, the words that came out of my mouth were not what I felt. I told Brian I had to take care of Mother, and because I had to focus on her, I could not marry him.

He just sat looking at me in shock. The pain in his eyes cut through me like a knife but I could not let it show on my face. Oh God, the pain in his eyes. Maybe that is why I just remembered this conversation. He walked over to me, knelt down, and told me No! He said he was not giving up on us. I told him it was not because I did not love him. Brain knew Daniel went to dialysis three times a week. But he didn't know what a struggle it was for me to pretend I was functioning like a normal woman. I had stopped being normal when I heard the diagnosis of Alzheimer's, but I didn't want him to know that. The woman he fell in love with was not the woman I was becoming.

When I finished talking, I took off my engagement ring and handed it to him. He started telling me how much he loved me and insisted he would always love me. Brian held my hand, looked me in the eye, and told me not to give up on us. He held me in his arms and said we would survive. I pulled away and asked him to please leave. He just sat there for what seemed like an hour.

I moved to a chair in the kitchen, my arms folded, not looking at him, waiting for him to leave. He asked me to sit with him but I refused. He kept telling me he loved me. I told him I knew he loved me, but it didn't matter, it couldn't matter. I could not nor would I marry him. He became angry. He begged me not to do this and asked me to think about what I was doing to us. I knew he did not understand. I felt I was right about this. He insisted he understood what I was going through, said our love would withstand anything. He pulled me into his arms and asked me not to let go of us. With every bit of strength I had, I gently pulled myself away from him and told him I did not need his help. I looked him in the eyes and asked him to please leave. I told him if he really loved me, he would leave me alone. Slowly he turned, walked to the door, placed the ring on the table, and left. As soon as the door closed and I knew he was gone, I cried uncontrollably. I cry today as I relive that day. I cry today. I cry.

Brian did not give up on me. I gave up on us. For days, weeks, and months, he would call or leave me flowers. He asked Daniel to talk to me. His parents called and left messages but I never returned their call. Daniel and I had bitter arguments. He wanted to know how I could love Brian and treat him as I did, but I never gave him an answer. Brian was persistent, but I would not return his calls or answer the door. I told my secretary not to accept calls from him. I screened all calls. I returned his letters and his flowers. I had to completely separate myself from him. I really wanted to believe he knew, deep down in his heart, that I made the right decision.

Weeks and weeks, then months and months went by until finally he gave up. I never heard from him again. I learned he moved back to England. Daniel and I never talked about Brian again.

Chapter 18

Daniel depended on me. He was not comfortable taking care of business matters, and I knew he did not feel capable of taking care of Mother by himself. He had to go to dialysis three times a week but for some reason, sometimes, would not go. He started drinking. I knew he was scared, frustrated, and felt his life was trapped, like mine. Daniel was not strong enough to handle what we were dealing with. I was the only one both of them could depend on.

I started to notice other changes in Mom. Whenever she stayed at my place in years past, she always had to get up at night but had no problem going to the bathroom. She slept on the side of my king-size near the bathroom, and I kept a night light on in the bathroom. Once I fall asleep, I sleep soundly.

One night I realized Mom had wet the bed. I was livid. I couldn't believe it—she did not get up! She was so ashamed and sincerely apologized. I calmed her down, gave her a shower, changed the sheets, and put her to bed. As I lay awake thinking about what had happened, I was so hurt for my mother. This was not like her. How could this be happening to my mother? I prayed to God it would not happen again. I asked, I begged Him to touch her mind with His healing power. And I finally cried myself to sleep.

The next morning I acted as if I was not too concerned about the night's event. But it stuck in my mind. I remember calling my brother at work. He said he would keep an eye on Mother. We felt we had resolved that issue. We had already refused to let her drive anymore. Now she could not keep track of time very well, she wet the bed, and she needed help dressing. Daniel continued to stay with her during the day, cooking and cleaning (looking back, I can only imagine his struggles to accept or comprehend his mother's situation).

For Mom all this was confusing, upsetting, and very unreal. Many times, I watched her become frustrated because she could not remember what day it was. I saw the fear in her eyes. She tried to make some sense of what was happening to her. She tried desperately to maintain her dignity and pride. She would be ashamed at times and asked us to forgive when she tried to remember how to cook dinner. We would reassure her—we understood, and things were okay.

My brother and I were scared but neither of us would admit it. And remember, we were not inviting anyone into our world. We could only wonder what challenges lay ahead. It is terrible to watch your mother, who has taken care of you from birth, given you advice and guidance all your life, and now she is mentally confused, yet still physically well. It is inconceivable.

These were uncharted waters. Daniel and I never had to really take care of anyone. We did not have children. All our lives we had depended on advice, encouragement, and sometimes even financial support from our parents. Now the roles were being reversed. The change was happening sadly, slowly and without our permission. I don't mean Daniel or I resented it, but we never imagined this could happen to us. To have to take care of our parents is not something any of us plans. I didn't want to be my mother's mother. Daniel and I needed a plan. We always expected to have to do something, but not this. We never, ever, expected to go through what we finally had to go through.

Chapter 19

Daniel and I had to make even more adjustments in our lives. Instead of going home after work, I went by Mother's every day. I gathered up the dirty laundry and took it home with me. I cleaned her house once a week. Daniel decided he would stay with Mother more often during the day, so I felt she would be safe. He was on dialysis and didn't work. If she needed to go anywhere, Daniel drove her. And he shopped for groceries. She was very comfortable with that arrangement; it made her feel secure. I scheduled her regular medical appointments and Daniel took her to them. She no longer trusted her judgment, so we were always there to help make decisions.

I did not realize it until years later, but I was beginning to lose me. Taking care of Mother consumed me night and day. I lost all my ambition to do anything other than take care of her. It consumed my time and devoured my spirit. Like my brother, I too was becoming a caregiver twenty-four hours a day. I paid her bills. I paid my bills. I shopped for her as well as myself. Sometimes I would buy a suit in her size and one in my size just to make it simple. When I traveled on business, it was difficult to relax. I worried. I called Daniel every day to make sure they were okay.

One day while traveling, I called and Mother answered the phone. When I asked her where Daniel was, she said she had not seen him for two days. Even though I had spoken with him the day before, I panicked. I called his cell with no answer. I called the hospital to find out if he was there for dialysis, but they indicated he wasn't there. I called the administration office in the apartment building, and they said they had not seen him. Now I was going out of my mind. I called Mother again but this time she explained that she was confused and Daniel had gone to the store. I hung up the phone and cried. This was stress. Sometimes it was difficult to concentrate, but I managed without going out of my mind. As soon as I returned home, I went by her place to make sure she was okay. I didn't like this. I wanted my life back, but this was Mother.

I started looking on the Internet for information that could help me. I learned that I needed to make sure that legal matters were in order, including health issues. She already had funeral arrangements made. However, other matters needed to be addressed. Daniel did not want the responsibility, so I became the executor of Mother's estate in case anything happened. She gave me the power of attorney, which included health care (I promised her I would not keep her alive on a machine). She and I also went to the bank and created a joint account. I was overwhelmed at times but I had to keep going. At work, I kept pretending my life was great. Brian had already stopped calling me. The only person I could confide in was Daniel; we were in this together by ourselves.

Chapter 20

At ninety-eight years old, Dad still lived by himself. He did not have any physical problems, and his mind was like a steel trap. Every morning he took his walk, kept his weight to 169 lbs, and drove wherever he wanted to go in his black Cadillac. He loved Cadillac's. Every car he ever owned was a black Cadillac. Daniel and I loved to go with him to buy a new car. We would look at all types of cars and try to convince him to buy some other car. Nevertheless, no, we always rode home in a black Cadillac. Dad was a quiet man. When he was home, he was always busy in his workshop. We would hear him whistling or humming and know he was busy making something. He was a great carpenter, self-taught. His memory was incredible. He remembered things he did while growing up and his facts were always right. Whenever he and my uncle got together, they would talk about the good old days.

I would often ask him to tell the story of how he met Mother or what San Francisco was like when he moved there. Dad said the lower part of

Van Ness Avenue was a cow patch in 1940. At first, he lived on California Street and rode the cable car to Powell Street to go to work. One day, he said he noticed the cable car driver was a woman. From then on, he would sit in a seat where he could watch her work the controls. Dad said she was the most beautiful woman he'd seen and had real pretty legs. He said he told his brother, my Uncle Jack, that he was going to marry her. Dad said it took him a year but sure enough, he married her. Whenever Dad told that story, Daniel and I would always turn to Mother and ask her why it took so long. She'd always say she knew he was the one but he was slow. Both of them would start laughing.

Because of his age, I know he had lived through some difficult times in the South but he never talked about them. Instead, he talked about the good things in life. How could Dad be well and Mother have Alzheimer's? I didn't understand.

Three years later, in June 1996, Dad's health began to fail. He had been completely self-sufficient. He had no medical conditions other than sometimes his knees ached a little. In June, he started having shortness of breath. He was experiencing chest pain and had problems breathing and walking up the stairs. I told him he needed to get a checkup and scheduled an appointment.

Since he was a veteran of World War I, I took him to the VA Hospital. Yes, he was in World War I. Dr. Gray was his primary physician. The funniest thing happened when Dad was talking to other doctors. The first or second question they asked would be, "Mr. Harris, how old are you?" He would casually say, "Ninety-eight years old." Immediately you would see their eyes light up. I remember the first time he said his age in the emergency room. The expression on that doctor's face was priceless. First puzzled, and then perplexed, he looked at him as if Dad was mentally unstable. Dad had never looked his age. He looked to be sixty-nine years old.

Doctors were always in total disbelief about Dad's age. They would elevate their voice to repeat the question. "Mr. Harris, I said, "How old are you?" emphasizing *you* like Dad certainly didn't hear the question. First, he would ask them why they were yelling and then tell his age. Doctors would smile from ear to ear. Sometimes they looked at me as if Dad was delirious. I would smile and confirm the answer. One of the doctors called several other doctors in and asked them to guess his age. Thinking it was a joke, they would look at Dad, look at me, and say, with a smile, "Late sixties, early seventies." Then Dad's doctor would tell them his true age. Dad was amazing. He had this dry humor. He would say something without smiling that made you burst in to laughter.

The doctors in the emergency room prescribed medication to help slow his heart rate. He was given oxygen, made comfortable, and in a few hours was feeling much better. After all the tests and X-rays, they determined that his heart was tired. Because of his age, a heart transplant was out of the question, but the doctors felt medication could stabilize his condition, and it worked!

When the symptoms returned in early August, this time they admitted him. I asked him if he was in pain, and he said, "No." He said it was just uncomfortable to breathe. There were papers for him to sign. I helped, but when I got to the question about resuscitation, I was not prepared to answer. His choice was Do Not Resuscitate. I must have looked worried because he looked at me and told me not to worry.

Now I readjusted my schedule to include visiting Dad every evening in the hospital. After leaving Mother's, I would go to the hospital, sit with him, and we would talk for hours. I loved listening to Dad tell me stories about growing up and what he did when he was young. We always ended our conversations talking about Mother. I knew he still loved her. He always smiled when he talked about how they met, and how she spurned his advances before accepting a date. Dad said the only regret he had in life was that he smoked cigars for a few years. One time we were laughing about something and he looked at me and said, "Take care of your mother; you know she's not all there." We both smiled. We were so close that even when there were problems we would always find something to laugh about.

For me, who had never had to visit a parent in the hospital before, this experience had been a rude awakening. I understood taking Dad to the hospital for an appointment, but for him to have to stay was unthinkable. The three of us had a new routine. On the days when Daniel didn't have dialysis, he and Mom visited Dad. After church on Sundays, we would visit him. Then we would go to Mother's and eat dinner.

When we drove to the hospital after church one Sunday, Dad had been there two weeks. As Mother, Daniel, and I walked down the hall to Dad's room, a nurse beckoned to us. We stopped and turned to see what she wanted. She said she had called me but was unable to reach me. I looked at my cell phone and realized I had not turned it back on after church. I apologized, but she looked at me and said she was sorry to tell us, but Dad had passed away.

Sunday, August 22, 1996. Dad is one month away from his ninety-ninth birthday. Something just punched me in the stomach. I cannot breathe. What did she say? Shock, disbelief, loss, bewilderment, fear, paralysis, hurt, and sadness, all these feelings hit me at once. There are no words to describe what happened next. But I'd talked to him before I went to church. There was always four of us and now three? We knew each other so well. We were close, very close.

I backed up to a wall, trying to get away from her words. I slid down the wall and not until I fell to the floor could I breathe. I wanted to scream. I did scream, but I could not hear myself. It would not come out. Or did it come out? I don't know. Daniel walked away. I saw him leaving but I could not respond. A nurse walked after him. He stopped walking and was escorted to a chair. I looked up and saw another nurse have Mother sit down. People were helping me to a chair. They tried to console us as best they could.

I don't remember how long we were there but I heard someone ask, "Did we want to see him?" I was in a daze. My brain was …numb. I have never seen a dead body in my life. I wanted to see him. I was scared. What would he look like? I asked the nurse and she told me he looked like he was asleep. He just passed away in his sleep. Mother was crying but suddenly she took over. Mother knew what we were talking about and, incredibly, she insisted she wanted to see him. We agreed. That moment gave us the strength to believe she was okay. She led us into the room and there he was. Dad was lying in bed as if he was asleep.

There were no tubes, no oxygen, just him lying there quietly, no breathing. Mother touched his brow and smiled. She leaned down and whispered something in his ear.

Years later, she admitted she told him she loved him and would always love him. I sat in the chair and watched as tears ran down my face. I could not touch him. How sad, I couldn't touch him, my own dad. I was scared, in shock, but I just couldn't touch him. I wanted him to be alive. I could not stop crying. Daniel stood by the bed and just looked at him. There had always been times when he was nonverbal, and this was one of those times. What a helpless feeling. We stayed for what seemed like an eternity, but it was probably only thirty minutes. We drove home in silence. Each of us trying to rationalize what had happened, and process what we were going to do now.

The days following my dad's death were very difficult to live through. Make the arrangements fell on my shoulders. I did not have time to be in shock. I had things to do. I called his pastor, my pastor, and Mother's pastor. My heart was broken, but I had to take charge and get things done. I was on remote control. I did what I had been told to do. That had been drilled into me for years. I called the appropriate people and made sure everything went as planned. There wasn't time to grieve.

When people tell you, "I know what you're going through," they mean it. But your relationship with your family is unique, just as my relationship with my family is unique. People think they know but they do not. At some point during the week, I did not want to hear one more person say, "I know what you're going through." I did not want to hear that any more. No one knows but you, and there is never closure. The best thing to say is my prayers are with you. That is it. I say that because I started resenting people telling me they knew how I felt. Trust me, *you don't know*!

Even now, as I write these words, I realize how important Dad was in my life. I depended on his guidance and his wisdom for so many years. When I had a problem I could call Dad, and in his special way, with dry humor, he would give me the answer.

Not only was I trying to cope with the

absence of Dad, whom I loved so dearly, but the full responsibility of taking care of Mother and Daniel was definitely on my shoulders. I took care of business. Sometimes Mother's memory would fade and she wouldn't remember Dad had passed away. I kept her with me that week. I completed the programs, ordered the flowers, called the minister, set the date and time, got the picture, picked the suit, consoled my brother, ordered the limo, contacted the cemetery, carried out Dad's instructions to the funeral home, etc. For the next week and a half, that was my task. Damn my own job!

My family was in crisis and that meant more to me than a job. I wanted to call Brian so many times, but I just could not force myself to do so. As far as I knew, Daniel was holding up well. He was not a talker, and sometimes he would just sit down and say nothing for hours.

When Aunt Willie passed away, it was not my responsibility to clean her house and remove her things; I left that for my cousin. However, with Dad, I had to empty his apartment and I was not prepared for that. Daniel and I decided to put that off until after the funeral. I spoke with my boss and explained that I would not return to work for several weeks.

At first, my boss seemed to understand, but after the third week, she insisted I needed to return to work soon. My priority was my family—I could always get a job. That is how I felt.

Not until the funeral service was over and we were at the gravesite did I finally realize Dad was gone. When we were emptying his apartment, everything became final. There should be a book somewhere explaining how to clean the house of a deceased family member. That was the worst ever.

So many times, I cried uncontrollably, and thought I would never stop. I would look at a chair or hear a voice that sounded like Dad's, and tears would begin to fall down my cheeks. There were times when I wasn't aware I was crying. I remember someone at work told a joke, a funny joke, I laughed, and suddenly I was crying without any explanation. It was so strange. When parents die, no matter what age you are, overwhelming and bizarre things begin to happen.

My most profound feeling of loss came

when I realized that Dad, the person I had depended on all my life, was no longer there. I could not call him anymore. That was a shocked and lonely feeling. As old as I was, I always had Dad. Part of me was gone. This now started THE FIRST. We all know THE FIRST. It begins on the next holiday, the next event, the next birthday, and any other next. The first time we go through a special occasion without our loved one. Life changes us. Somehow, for me THE FIRST STILL GOES ON AND ON AND ON.

Both Father's and Mother's Day were our family days. After Sunday morning services on his day we would take Dad to his favorite restaurant, Sizzler's. He got cards and gifts from each of us. I always called that morning and sang. Happy Father's Day to him like it was his birthday. After he passed, I had nothing. No Dad to be with. And it really hurt. Even though I was a grown woman, watching other people with their father was hard.

To compound my pain, I was literally watching Mother slowly disappear. It was not a physical absence but a mental disappearance, which was even worse. I was becoming the mother and she was slowly becoming the child. Oh God, this pain was so much more than that of a quick death. The confusion, the unknown, the uncertainty were overwhelming. Not only do you watch them disappear but you too are disappearing. The essence of who you were is slowly going away. Your hopes, dreams, life, loves are no longer important. You take a backseat to your ailing loved ones and you don't even realize it.

For almost a year, Daniel and I took care of Mother alone. We were in denial. Both of us hoped, prayed, and waited for things to get better. I needed a miracle. I thought if I didn't accept what was happening, somehow it wouldn't happen. We also didn't want anyone else to know what was happening. We were not ashamed; we were just very private people.

Going to church, every Sunday was important to Mother. She had always looked elegant and dressed like a lady, so I made sure her appearance did not change. Before leaving, she would look in the mirror and smile, pleased. Every other Sunday Daniel would take her to her church, just across the street. I was proud to have him as my brother. To give him a break, I would take her to my church the other Sundays.

For me, weekends presented another challenge and a change in my life's routine. Friday night I would pick Mother up and bring her to my place. Saturday became the girls' day out. I woke, prepared breakfast, dressed her, and we would go shopping. I made sure she got a manicure and pedicure, and sometimes a facial. I cooked dinner made sure she took a bath, and prepared her clothes for Sunday. Mother loved church services. On Sunday mornings, I would wake early enough to dress both of us, feed her breakfast, and make sure she took care of her physical needs.

This was not a new challenge. Mother had always been the one who had us stop on the road for bathroom breaks. I remember our trips to the ranch on Saturdays. Dad proclaimed that we would leave at 6:00 a.m. and would tell us to be ready. Daniel and I might wake up late, but by six o'clock, we were ready. Mother, on the other hand, would have been up since 4:00 getting our picnic basket ready, yet she was the last one to get in the car. She'd be in the house, cleaning. Mother always claimed that if anything ever happened, no one would come into our house and find it messy. Dad drove. By the time, we were nearing Sausalito (about 15 minutes from our house); she'd ask that all-important question. She would turn to him, smile, and say, "How close do you think the next service station is?" He would sigh. He knew that was her code word indicating she needed a bathroom stop. We always made two stops before we got to the ranch, that's just the way it was. We were used to the question.

Now Mom had Alzheimer's, and one of the things we had to know when we went shopping with her was where the bathrooms were located. When she would look at me and ask, "Do you think they have a bathroom?" I knew what that meant. There was a need, and I had to find one fast. Nail salons always had bathrooms, but many stores do not have them for customers.

As Mom's condition progressed, she would sometimes ask that question very late, which did not allow much time to find one. On several occasions, we had dressed and were walking to the car when she needed to return to the house. Sometimes when Daniel and I were together, just trying to relax, we would share stories of our adventures with Mother. If something happened to him, I knew it would happen to me when she was in my care. We laughed at the challenges Mother took us through.

One time Daniel and Mother went shopping at Safeway and she proclaimed she had to go. Being a man, he did not know what to do. He asked a checker and, sure enough, Safeway had a public bathroom. Who knew? That was something neither of us had ever considered when shopping for groceries. Once she finished, they continued shopping.

But then while they were at the checkout stand, suddenly he had to go. We laughed so hard. He said he now had the same problem of looking for bathrooms while shopping; it was rubbing off on him. We laughed about that for years, because sure enough, the same problem devolved on him. When I was with the two of them, they wore me out. Never did both of them want to go at the same time, so we just made adjustments. I made sure to scout the area for bathrooms whenever I went out with them, just because.

When I took Mother to my church, I would

make sure she sat where I could observe her. She enjoyed services, as I said. Life was changing for both of us but it was still manageable on Sunday nights. Taking her back to her place after church was difficult, though. She enjoyed staying with me, and I enjoyed having her, but I could not take a chance on leaving her at my place by herself. Like a child, she would be very persistent in wanting to stay with me, but my decision was based on both our needs. I had to go to work

Daniel would be waiting for her at her place, so that helped convince her to go home. Once I got her undressed, bathed, and bedded, I would go back to my apartment. I'd relive the weekend in my head and feel good about what I did. Or if Mother called me once she was home, she calmed down only when I reassured her she'd be with me the next weekend. It was very sad.

I know she understood life was changing, and we wanted to keep as much order in her life as possible. Having a routine sustained her for years. She knew Daniel would stay with her, and she knew I would call at least four or five times a day to check on her. I did not take vacations. If I took time off work, I used that time to rest. Or I would clean both of our apartments.

Taking care of Mother and working began to take a toll. While necessary, work was becoming less important. My attitude was affecting my concentration. My primary responsibility had shifted to caring for Mother.

It was just a job; it was not my life, my career. I worked to get a paycheck, to pay the bills. I could always get another job, but I could not get another Mother. She became the focus of my life. I used to spend Saturdays and evenings painting abstracts in oil, but I had not thought of anything like that or wanted to do it for years. Dating was not going to happen. No time.

Both of us were fighting to keep the essence of our identity and losing the battle. We chose different ways to cope. I was always searching the Internet for anything that could help me understand what I needed to do in order to keep Mother safe and maybe, just maybe, find some medicine to help reverse this condition. I read about the research, but there was no cure. I even looked for alternative medicines to remedy the condition.

Daniel, on the other hand, never gave up trying to keep his life normal, separate. There were times when I thought he was at home with Mother only to find out he was not. That scared me. And I noticed that he drank a little more. He was not interested in getting a kidney transplant. I kept mentioning it to him, but he never really seemed to care. He just accepted dialysis as his lifestyle.

Finally, I realized that we needed outside help. I can't remember when I first heard about the food delivery program for seniors, but it was a Godsend. The food was prepared and sent to the house in nice containers. They'd deliver Monday through Saturday. And on Saturday, they'd deliver an additional meal for Sunday. Yes! This revelation would free Daniel and me from cooking.

We called and started the service. The challenge now was to get Mother to open the door for this strange person to deliver these meals. We asked them to have the same person deliver the meals. This gave her some comfort, and I wouldn't have to go by her place every day. Daniel moved in with his girlfriend, so we both felt a little relief. I still called four or five times a day, to make sure she was okay and had received and eaten the meals; that could also be a problem. She ate them. I was relieved. We were feeling good about this.

Then during one of my visits, I found she had stored all the food in the refrigerator and was not eating. Another setback and another challenge—a new problem had surfaced. This lady from Hattiesburg Mississippi was used to red beans and rice, hot water cornbread, succotash, fried chicken and pork chops. She was not accustomed to eating tortellini. Other dishes, while good, were unfamiliar to her, and she simply refused to eat them. I had to discontinue the meal service because I found meals in the trash or in the refrigerator uneaten.

I asked around and found another food service for seniors in her community that catered primarily to African-Americans. It was only two blocks from her place. I ran, not walked, to sign Mother up. When I told Daniel about the center, it was like Christmas for both of us. This was a GOOD thing. The foods were familiar to her and I knew she would eat them. I was there when they delivered her first meal and introduced her to the deliveryman. He delivered all her meals so she was not afraid to answer the door for him. This lasted for a few months. I started to notice she was now eating smaller portions. Daniel and I were concerned. Mother no longer had a good appetite.

Mother also had a ritual of getting dressed, walking to McDonald's (which was located on the corner), and getting breakfast. This was her morning routine. If she was not at home, I knew she would be at McDonald's restaurant. She tried to keep that routine, which now really scared me.

I had put off buying her a cell phone—worried she'd lose it—but this forced me to purchase one. I had to keep in constant touch with her. Luckily, my job was in San Francisco. I often used lunchtime to go to her place just to make sure she was safe. I finally decided to let the apartment manager know about Mother's condition. She said she understood, especially since there were other senior residents in the building with memory problems. She agreed to try to keep an eye on Mother if she ever saw her on the street. That gave me a little comfort. I knew I had to have someone closely monitor her movement.

Overwhelmed! That is what I felt like. I was overwhelmed! I was so involved sometimes that I forgot to pay my own bills. I worried all the time. Trying to keep a routine was difficult. Many a time I panicked at work. I might call her and not receive an answer. I'd leave my job, rush over to her place to make sure nothing drastic had happened. And often I'd find she was still in bed, even though it would be 12:00 or 1:00. I'd get her dressed and have her eat something. Of course, that would happen on the days my brother had dialysis.

I would stay with her until Daniel came back. Many nights I stayed awake trying to plan her week and my week around my brother's dialysis schedule. This lasted for several years.

I finally accepted that she needed someone to care for her during the day. I asked Social Services to assign a worker to assist her and to make sure her place stayed clean. But I was apprehensive. To allow a perfect stranger into the house is scary enough for me, but for Mother I knew it might be impossible. Imagine you know your mind is not functioning as well as it has all your life. In addition, a strange person is coming into your home, going through your things.

The position really was impossible. Mother could not accept strangers in her house. She became argumentative and angry. The anger was not really toward me or at the worker. She was feeling helpless, and I was the one who took her verbal abuse. I understood, I really did, but it hurt. Something had to change. (I had heard stories about Alzheimer's patients wandering off and could no longer take the chance of her getting lost. I bought her a bracelet with her name and phone number on it, just in case.)

Some workers would last two days. Another one lasted a week. One day I made a surprise visit only to find Mother still in bed. She also had not been fed. I was enraged. I wanted to stuff that worker in the garbage can and shoot her. Instead, I fired her. I suddenly realized that not all caregivers are in the profession to help; some are in the business just for the money. I made a vow to myself to make sure that anyone who took care of Mom would treat her with the dignity and respect she deserved.

I knew Daniel would really get out of

control if anyone mistreated her. I didn't want him to go to jail, so I never told him why I fired the last worker. This consumed my thoughts and I knew I had to find an alternative.

Chapter 21

I needed an alternative and needed it fast. I was not comfortable leaving Mother isolated at home. I was afraid to take a chance with strangers. When I was at work, I had to concentrate and do my job. It was my escape. I couldn't take the chance of something happening while I was away on business. I refused to attend many important meetings that could have advanced my career. I never planned a vacation.

I cannot remember when, where, or how I learned about adult day care. But I wanted Mother in it. I visited the Senior Center. The staff seemed caring and professional. Seniors of all ages were there for the day. They were served breakfast and lunch and encouraged to participate in arts, crafts, and exercises to help stimulate their minds. A van would pick Mom up and take her to the facility. She would spend the day with seniors who had the same condition she had. At 3:00 p.m., the van would return her to her place. This was great. Yes, I had found the answer.

Daniel and I planned how this could work. He scheduled his dialysis from 11 to 1:00 so he could help her dress to make sure she got on the van. By the time she was due to come home, one of us would be there to meet the van to make sure she got home safely. I changed my schedule at work. Yes, we could manage this. I would not have to worry about her during the day. She would be free and the activities would stimulate her brain. She could get better. Yes. That is what we wanted. I immediately signed her up.

We sat her down and explained what was going to happen. I really felt she understood what we said. Day care was to start on Monday.

A few years had passed since we started this journey. My life had changed. Friends I used to call regularly, I had not spoken to them for a long time. They would call, but I had no time to chat with them. I stopped participating in other activities. I could not remember the last time I went to the movies. I stopped thinking about trying to paint a long time ago. I cannot remember the last time I read a book. I just did not have the energy anymore. Dully, I recognized a familiar pattern of mine. Once I got home, I headed for bed. That was my refuge. That was my escape. I turned on the TV, watched for a while, and then fell asleep. I never really saw any shows because I was numb. You know that feeling when you just stare at the TV screen. Time passes, but if anyone asked you what you saw, you have no memory of it. Well that's how I was.

I was numb. I was disconnected from life. Now that I think about it, I was disconnected for a long time. In fact, I could not remember when it happened. Maybe the reality of what I was going through put me in that room in my mind. Like Mother, I was putting myself, the essence of me, in a mental room. I stopped caring about my life. I never fought for me. I gave over to the circumstances around me and reacted to what was happening to everyone else but me. I never really grieved over the loss of my dad. I missed him tremendously. I just never had the time to grieve. I missed the mental image I had made as a child—my parents together, taking care of each other. That is what was supposed to happen. I was supposed to be married and taking care of my own kids. Well, I did not have time to think about all that; I had to get up and make sure Mother did not miss the van.

On that first day, I arrived at her house at

least one hour before the van was due. She was happy to see me. I got her up, washed, and dressed without a problem. She did not remember our talk about the Day Care. She thought I was there because it was Saturday, our day. Daniel and I kept telling her about the van and what she was going to do that day. That's when the argument began. She insisted she was not going because she could take care of herself. We insisted. She finally agreed to go downstairs.

Getting her in the van with strangers was our next challenge. How was I going to do it? I told her she would have fun. I told her the bus was for seniors only and I could not go with her. When she insisted, I told her I would pick her up, which calmed her down. This was a lie. We knew she was scared and she got on the bus reluctantly. Some of the other seniors were in wheelchairs. They looked sickly. Not Mom. She had her purse; she was dressed the way she liked to look. When they sat her down and put her seat belt on, she calmed down. I reminded her that the van would bring her home. She stopped complaining. I quickly went to my car and followed the van, crying all the way.

I observed from a distance. I needed to know she was going to be okay, for her sake and for mine. After about half an hour, I decided to go into the facility but I didn't go in the room where the seniors were located. I looked through the door of the large room but stayed out of sight, so Mother would not see me. Some of the seniors were in a circle, in wheelchairs, others like Mother in regular chairs. They were being given breakfast. Some had orange juice, some milk, and a few, like Mother, were drinking coffee. She did not appear confused, but she was very apprehensive.

I noticed they had a piano and introduced myself to the manager, asking if Mother could play while she was there. The manager was delighted and said yes. We also talked about the activities. After breakfast, people would be given some exercise classes and other activities. Unlike me, Mother believed in exercise (I was not an exercise person even though I really needed it more than she did. I stopped taking care of me a long time ago).

When the manager introduced herself to Mother, I saw her smiling and knew everything would be all right. I left. As I got into my car, I felt hopeful. This would work. Thank God. I called Daniel and told him how well it went. We both rejoiced. This event was a milestone on our amazing journey. There would finally be some stability in all our lives.

Months passed. On several occasions, Daniel would do a disappearing act, and for a few days, I could not find him. Then he would reemerge as if nothing had happened. He was not as strong as I was. I had built up a wall. I was tough. My emotions were in check. I did what I had to do.

I continued my duties as both overseer and daughter. I felt we could function on this level forever. It would last for many years, and I could keep my sanity. I prayed to God that Mother would not get any worse, no matter what the doctors said.

I interacted with those who were taking care of Mother. While I still didn't focus on my individual needs, I functioned. I worked until I was tired, then retreated to my place, and immediately went to bed. There was nothing else. As far as anyone looking at me was concerned, I was okay.

In retrospect, I realize, I was depressed beyond belief. I didn't have time to take care of me.

I was the oldest. I had to make sure Daniel went to his treatments even when he did not want to. I had to make sure that there were clean clothes, and Mother was dressed nicely.

Now that I am writing this, I remember something that my mother loved to do. Her most favorite thing was to chew gum. She loved Double mint. She had to have that before going to bed. I never wanted her to run out. I made sure a pack of gum was in her nightstand by the bed. Of course, as her condition progressed, I would find wads of gum in the strangest places.

Daniel and I would laugh about where we would find gum. He said one night when he got up to go to the bathroom in the dark; he stepped on something as he entered the room. It scared him. He said at first he could not figure out what was stuck to his foot.

Chapter 22

A year and a half later, I was in a meeting, and there was a phone call from my brother. This was one of many calls; everyone in the office knew that if Daniel called there was a family problem. He sounded so distraught it scared me. Daniel was like Dad, he kept his emotions hidden. He had Dad's attitude at heart, or he gave the appearance of being strong. He said Mother was having a problem, and would I come to the house. I left work and drove to the house as fast as possible.

When I arrived, Mother was still in bed. I know she had not been eating much, but on this day I suddenly realized how small she was—as if her body was shrinking, as well as her mind. I asked her, "Why don't you want to go on the van?" She said, "What van?" "I don't remember any van." She asked me why she would have to go on a van. A pain hit in the pit of my stomach. Oh God, I thought. What am I going to do?

I stayed with her that day trying to snap her out of this. She asked me to take her to my place. We tried to explain why I couldn't. I had to work.

She couldn't function alone at my place. What could I do?

I thought about quitting my job and staying home to take care of Mother, but that was financially impossible. I called the Senior Center and told them she would not be coming that day. The next day she seemed better. We continued the van schedule again. Weeks passed.

Months later, I went on a business trip. When I returned home, Daniel said Mother tried to get out of bed and fell down. He said she did not hurt herself but I called an ambulance and had her taken to the hospital to make sure she hadn't broken any bones. They assured me she was physically very healthy. They suggested Mother be kept overnight for observation. And because she was a little dehydrated, they would give her an IV. I agreed to have her stay. During that time, she never got out of bed. She had stopped feeding herself or dressing herself. She had not been eating well. The doctor indicated that the dementia was causing this change, and he felt it might be time to place her in a nursing home. I talked to her, trying to convince her to get out of bed, but she didn't seem to understand what I was saying.

When I looked in her face and into her eyes, I realized something was missing. Mother was missing. The person I have known all my life was gone. That twinkle was gone. That light was gone. This person was no longer my mother. I was losing the battle but I vowed to fight for her until the end. I would bring her back.

I was able to find a nursing home that had a rehabilitations facility to help Mother walk again. I looked at many facilities, making surprise visits to see what they were like after visiting hours. Did they allow family members any time? How did the facilities look? I finally found one that was well maintained, very clean, and the workers were caring people. It had chandeliers and a beautiful dining room. There were daily activities for the patients and a piano in the dining room. I knew Mother would like it. Members of different churches would visit and have church services and small concerts. They had a rooftop seating area overlooking the city. And they had rehab. This was perfect. Mother would not need to stay long. The rehab employees were there for the sole purpose of helping patients gain strength, so they could return home. I wanted Mother restored. She would return home and start taking the van again. That was my plan.

I don't remember when I lost hope. Mother was never going to revert to the mother I knew again. I had needed that hope to keep me going. I needed the feeling that I was stopping this process. Once I realized I had no control over what was happening; I did not know how I would react. Only God could help me.

The hospital kept her under observation for two days. Afterward they would transfer her to the nursing home. This was the most devastating thing I had ever imagined. Never! NO! I could not do that! Not a nursing home. Never would I put Mother in a nursing home. Dear God, I prayed, please help me. There must be something else.

I cried until I had no more tears. I lost all my energy. I do not drink, but I bought a bottle of liquor, took it home, and drank it all. What could I do? Why was this happening? Why was Mother being punished? I asked God Why ME? Why HER?

Of all the decisions I ever had to make, the most painful one was to place Mother in a nursing home. There is no pain worse than the feeling I had that last day. Daniel and I packed up her clothes. In between crying and taking her to the bathroom, I helped get Mother dressed.

I was having an out-of-body experience that day. Knowing it had to be done did not help me. I wanted to be rich so that I could take care of her properly. I was giving up. I was throwing her away. I put myself in her place and could not imagine this being done to me. As I write this, I cry. The pain of that day haunts me to this day. Did I do the right thing? Wasn't there something else I could have done? I will take that feeling with me to my grave. I know it was best for her but if I could have done anything else in this world, I would have. Was I a bad daughter? Were we bad children?

As we entered Mother's room, she looked so frail and small. She recognized Daniel and me. I kissed her on the cheek and we talked. The attendants came to prep her for the move. She asked if she was going home with me. My mouth was dry. I had no words. Again, I explained to her what was going to happen. She was going to a nursing facility to help her walk again. They put her in the ambulance. Daniel rode with her and I followed in my car. The nurses at the rehab facility greeted us and introduced themselves. She was gracious and polite to them. When we arrived on the floor where she was to stay, they had prepared a bed for her next to the window. She had a view of the city. I asked her if she felt like sitting in the wheelchair for a while. She said she was tired and wanted to lie down.

This was my last hope. If she had only been able to make an attempt to get up and walk, this experience was over. I would take her home and continue my vigil. They picked her up and put her in bed. The nurses brought over a wheelchair and told her if she wanted to get up the chair was there to help her get around. She smiled and thanked them. I put her things away and sat down by her bed. The other ladies in the room introduced themselves, and she suddenly realized something was very different.

Mother asked if I was taking her home with me, I tried to talk but nothing came out. Daniel tried to explain. I could only nod my head, no. Once she started walking again, I said, I would have her live with me. I meant that! Daniel left the room.

Dad's death was not as painful as what I felt that day. If you have ever had to go through this process then you know what I mean. No words can explain the feeling, the emotions, the hurt, the guilt, and the shame you feel leaving your mother at a nursing home alone.

It had been eight years since we started this process. I looked at my mother, my little mother, and I knew this was not what she expected to happen. She could never have imagined being in a situation where she had no control of her mind, body, and spirit. I know she would never have wanted her life end in such an uncontrollable situation. Imagine that you have the physical capability of putting on your clothes, but you cannot remember how it's done. Mother was fading from me and I couldn't stop it.

After a few weeks, Mother stopped talking. She would acknowledge my presence with a smile, but she just stopped talking completely.

Every day for several months, Mother was wheeled upstairs for a rehabilitation sessions. She was not progressing. Each time I got off the elevator, I remember, I hoped that Mother would be walking toward me, and that this nightmare would be over.

One day I was asked to meet with a therapist to discuss her progress. As always, the therapist was polite, but I knew it was not going to be a good conversation. I could see it on his face. He explained that in Mother's case, because she had not walked in months and now had stopped talking, in his professional opinion she would never walk again. I was crushed. He had discussed her progress with the other therapists, and they had not seen any improvement. He tried to reassure me, this was the normal progression of the disease. I realized this was not something he wanted to tell me, but I had to know. He would no longer have her brought up to rehab.

I was losing hope. I knew he was right. As I walked toward her, she smiled. I smiled. I couldn't let her see my disappointment. I wanted to keep her spirits up. I wheeled her to the rooftop and sat down. I talked to her, still asking her questions and hoping she would answer. The view of the city was beautiful, but my heart was breaking. She enjoyed having the sun on her face. I talked to her for about an hour. It was nearing time for dinner, so I took her to the dining hall where she ate a little. It was becoming difficult to get her to eat. She just was not interested in eating anymore. I was worried. I had a long talk with the doctor who indicated this was part of the condition. I hate this! To avoid her having to be force-fed I strongly encouraged her to eat.

I now did all the talking, but Mother would show her feelings by the expression. I combed her hair, took her to the bath, and got her dressed for bed. Lifting her was not easy, but I wanted to know if I could do it without a problem. I quickly realized that even though she had lost weight, she was still heavy to carry. I could not manage to get her into bed by myself. I called for a nurse to help me, and we got her in bed safely. I tucked her in and she smiled. I knew then she realized I was doing the best I could. She was thankful. Sometimes her smile really helped me accept this challenge. She wasn't angry. Mother always had a sweet disposition. She closed her eyes and was drifting off to sleep when I left.

Once I got in the car, I could not hold it in any longer. I sat there and cried. Once I regained my composure, I drove home and went immediately to bed. I needed to make another painful decision. If Mother was not going to get better, I needed to relinquish her apartment. I had to decide what to do with her things. I already had Dad's things, and now I would need to decide what to do with Mom's belongings. I knew she could never stay by herself again.

The next day I called Daniel. Since he had given up his apartment to stay with Mother, I knew this was going to be a challenge for him as well. He would move in with his girlfriend permanently. We had to decide what to do with her furniture, clothes, etc. I had enough furniture but we took a few pieces as we did when Dad passed. The remaining furniture was appraised and sold. After the movers left, I just sat in the empty apartment and cried. I seemed to be crying a lot. Daniel tried to comfort me. We decided we had to accept what was happening.

Mother never asked to come to my place again. I believe in her heart she realized she was not going to get better and had accepted it. Mother was very spiritual. I visited every day but it was so hard. I would bring her flowers, sit, and read to her. I would still take her to the rooftop, sit, and enjoy the sun. However, it wasn't the same anymore. The nurses indicated she still was not eating her meals, as she should. She was very, very small.

I met with the doctor and he indicated at this stage of her condition sometimes patients were given nourishment through an IV. I agreed to the IV but tried to get her to eat. It was frustrating trying to feed her, but eventually she would eat. I explained to her that I did not want her to have to be force-fed, but if she did not eat, I would have to make that decision. She would eat a little more. Daniel and his girlfriend visited Mom in the evenings, also trying to convince her to eat.

Chapter 23

It had been almost six months since she became bedridden. That day I came in, she was just lying in bed and looking out of the window. I spoke to her and she smiled. She finally spoke to me and whispered that she had seen her sister. I was astonished. I said, your sister. She whispered yes.

I could not speak anymore. Words would not come. I had a lump in my throat. I am a spiritual person myself. Yes, I knew what she meant. She spoke to me. Tears rolled down my cheek. She knew me. I was so glad.

I raised the head portion of the bed. I still could not speak. I combed her hair and braided it. I asked her, "When did you see your sister?" She never responded, just smiled. I took her frail hands and started putting nail polish on her nails. I knew she liked that. I massaged her arms and legs. I still could not speak. She kept smiling. I was not the only person she was smiling at. It was as if she was smiling at people around me and beyond me.

I sat with her for hours not saying anything.

I was scared. I was so overwhelmed. In my heart, I knew she was leaving me for good. Daniel came in at about 10:00 p.m. I was surprised because it was so late. For some reason, he insisted he was going to stay the night, which was very unusual. I believe he felt the same way I did that day.

I could not stay. I kissed Mother. She gripped my hand and smiled. It was her way of telling me she loved me, and that she was okay. I wanted to run and scream but I couldn't.

I don't remember the drive home. When I closed the door, all I could do was to sit in a chair in a daze. Hours later Daniel called me, crying, and told me Mother had passed.

I knew it. I cried so much that I could not cry anymore. I never went to bed. I called the mortuary. Daniel stayed with Mother until the funeral home came to get her. I couldn't do it. I just could not go there and watch them take my mother to the funeral home. Daniel was strong. My brother waited.

Chapter 24

Once again, I knew what to do. I went to the funeral home and waited until they arrived. Mother had talked to me about this for years; she drilled it in my head. I knew what to do. I told them what happened and they took over. All I had to do was to take the papers to them. I knew what she wanted to wear. I made sure her instructions were followed.

The service was beautiful. She was dressed in a white suit with a rose in hand. White limo, white dress, and white roses. And I wore white. I sang her favorite song like she told me to do. We carried ourselves in a dignified manner. There was no screaming, wailing, throwing ourselves on the casket.

I don't remember the ride to the cemetery or how I got home. I know I was empty, numb, and confused. There was no need for me to act. I did everything for her when she was alive. She was at peace. I had no regrets about that. To others I was a rock, while inside I died.

Chapter 25

The worst part of losing a loved one is that you stay. They do not have to suffer anymore, and that is a good thing. You, you have to go through the process after they pass away and that is worst.

People always say, "I know what you're going through, because my mother passed away too." While that may sound sympathetic, and I am not saying you should not comfort someone, no one in the world knows what you are going through. Your relationship with your loved one was not theirs. It is yours. After hearing that sentiment from so many people, I began to hate it. I did not want to hear another person tell me that. I started to become angry and resentful. No one can understand someone else's grief.

Grief takes on many forms and makes us do many things. I went through days, weeks, and months in a haze. I did what people expected me to do. I acted as if I was together. I functioned in a somewhat stable way. I ate, slept, and for the most part, I was "normal." To others I was normal. The problem was that even though I thought I was functioning, I wasn't. Once Mother passed away, I had all this time on my hands. I had no place to go after work. I never needed to call the nursing home to ask how she was. I did not have to go by her place to clean it up. On Saturdays, I didn't know what to do. Even today, some Saturdays are still difficult. For months and months, my depression was most noticeable to me on Saturdays.

I just could not get out of bed. I had built my life around the activities with my mother for so long that when it she was gone there was a void in my life. I forced myself to try to get active. Eventually I would turn on the TV. I never watched it. I needed to hear noise. I rarely slept.

Daniel, my brother whom I loved so much, was having his own problems too. I don't know what it was like for him watching Mother pass away. He never talked about it and I never asked him. We tried to keep in touch with each other but it was difficult because now it seemed we really didn't have anything to talk about.

At the beginning, we tried to talk every day, but gradually we drifted apart. I think we needed the separation to try to get ourselves back to where we were. He and his girlfriend were trying to create a life of their own and I respected that. They moved out of the city. He would call me once or twice a week.

I was a recluse as far as outside activities go. I refused singing engagements. I was always busy when friends called to ask me out for dinner. I functioned outside my apartment, but inside I was numb. I no longer cared what it looked like. I neglected myself. On special occasions, I invited Daniel and his girlfriend for dinner, but it was difficult.

Eventually, he would cancel. I stopped cooking those big meals that Mother made. When Daniel came over, we would sit and talk, trying to act as if we were survivors. And we were. The only problem was that we did not know how to communicate in a non-crisis mode. Sometimes Daniel refused to go to dialysis. Several times his doctor called me asking if he was on his way. I would call his girlfriend and she would tell me he refused to go. Dialysis is critical when you have kidney failure. I would get so angry with him. Why would he not go? Failing to have dialysis put pressure on his other organs. He would have to go to the emergency to have an immediate dialysis. This happened too many times.

One Friday in January 2006, Daniel called me from the hospital to say he was going to have emergency dialysis. As usual, I gave him hell. He promised to change and told me he would call when he got home. He didn't call, but it was not unusual for him not to keep his word, so I did not worry.

I called him Saturday evening, but there was no answer. I called his girlfriend, but she said he was probably at his apartment. He always kept his apartment so that when they had a fight, he had a place to go. Sunday morning I called and failed to receive an answer. I then called the front desk and asked them to knock on Daniel's door. I knew when he slept sometimes it was hard to get him to wake up. The clerk told me there was no answer at the door. I gave him verbal permission to go into his apartment and to call me back. I waited for over an hour.

I had just decided to drive over to his apartment when the phone rang. The caller asked me if I was alone. I said, "Yes, why"? He said that he was sorry to tell me but that my brother, Daniel, was dead.

Dead! What do you mean, Dead! That's all I heard. I don't remember anything else. My mind stopped processing information. I know I dropped the phone and screamed. Dead! Daniel. Dead. No, this could not be happening. Daniel was all I had left.

I told them to call an ambulance because he could not be dead and I was coming there. I drove like a wild person, double-parked behind the ambulance, ran into the apartment building. Two police officers held me back. Their faces told me the whole story. It was true. Daniel was dead.

Oh God! No! Again I went through the process of calling a funeral home, arranging funeral services, picking the clothes, paying the bills, giving the clothes away, getting rid of furniture, going to the cemetery, the stuff, the stuff, the stuff you have to do to bury your loved ones, the stuff. After Mother died, it took me four months before I could go back to work. After Daniel died, it took me another four months.

Chapter 26

If you watched me, I acted like I was a normal, functioning person. This went on for more than a year. Actually, it went on for more than three years before I realized I had to make a serious change. I thought about a therapist but I felt there was nothing anyone could tell me that I didn't already know. I knew I needed to snap out of it. I knew I needed to move on with my life. I did not need a stranger to tell me that. I didn't need to medicate myself to cause new problems. What I needed to do was to make a change.

Everything and everybody I saw reminded me of what life was before my family passed away. Where I lived, people I saw all reminded me of what I loss. Even smells began to bring back memories. Everything was too much of a reminder. I made a change in my life, and that is how I am making a grief recovery.

While you may not believe it, your surroundings can affect your recovery. Make a change. Change where you live. Change how you live. De-clutter. Change where you work. Change how you work. Change your hairstyle. Look at what you can do to your living surroundings. Join a gym. Take a walk! Go out and do it!

Do SOMETHING! Just make a change. The new experience will focus you on starting a new life. You will begin to enjoy who you are. That is how I was finally able to finish this book. My memories are vivid some days. I still have the urge to pick up the phone and call Mother, Dad, or Daniel. Grief will always be with me. Your mind does not just let it go, it holds onto it. You need to remember your past because it affects your future. The change made it not so painful.

Remember the good times, the good days. When I see the elderly now, I am more conscious of what they may be feeling. I wonder what they may be going through. When I hear that someone's relative has Alzheimer's or any kind of illness, I pray for him or her. I cannot guess to know what they are going through, but I feel their pain. I tell them I will be praying for them and their recovery and I do.

Life is short. What we do and what we are

affects others in so many ways. A kind word or deed will help; you and you will feel better too.

I hope this book helps you understand that while my mother's illness was shattering and heartbreaking, it made me become who I am today. It made me a stronger, more caring human being. Remember, grief does not always end. If it does for you, then you are truly blessed. There is a hole in my heart. But I stay busy and have become more creative.

This book was my aid to recovery. While writing this book, I opened many locked-up memories of who I was and what I liked. It helped me remember what I loved about life. It helped to ease the pain but it will not go away. We all grieve about something. We are all hurting. Love yourself enough to give yourself permission to hurt and still have happiness. We all make adjustments to survive. Hurting others won't heal you.

I don't make my expectations of others too high, and if they let me down, I pray for them. My spirit is much more tolerant than before. I allow myself to enjoy the moment. I no longer criticize others, because I do not know what they are going through. We are all in pain on some level. Physically, mentally, spiritually we are all in need of something or someone.

I know how to be happy. I am happy to wake up in the morning. I laugh aloud at commercials. I enjoy me all by myself. I live one day at a time.

If you want to heal, smile! Keep going! You will make it. Would my family have wanted me to tell this story? Yes! They lived life helping others. Maybe someday you can tell somebody your story and it can help someone else. Smile. If you do nothing but smile, it will make you feel better.

He will yet fill your mouth with laughter; And your lips with rejoicing.

(Job 8:21)

Afterword

Being a caregiver is not always a choice. For most of us, circumstances turn us into caregivers. We don't just decide one day that we want to be caregivers. I didn't. I admire those in the medical field because they choose their profession. Me, I had no other choice.

Mother didn't choose to have Alzheimer's, but because she had it, I had to become responsible for her. Assuming that role changed my life. I do not ever regret doing it; I just never dreamed I would be in that position. When I finally faced facts, I looked for a step-by-step book on what I needed to know. There wasn't one. I don't know if there can be one. Each of us has different circumstances and challenges—emotional, physical, financial, and environmental. There is no age restriction for caregivers. You may start the day a sibling is born with an unexpected health condition. You may start after you retire and find that your husband, sister, or parent needs care. You can't plan ahead.

When I was growing up, I made choices. I decided what I wanted to do in life. I decided how I would look, dress, eat, sleep, walk, talk, drive, shop, and cook. I decided whom I would date. Those choices were MY choices. A caregiver is robbed of that ability to choose. Your choices depend on the person you care for. Suddenly, you can't take a trip because your responsibilities now dictate your need to care for your loved one. Often there will be no one else but you. You stop thinking about a vacation or any other activity that will require your absence. Eventually, you give up even wanting to go away because you know, if you do, your thoughts will be consumed with what is happening back home.

Every one of us is dealing with something. Parents may have an autistic child. Sisters, brothers, aunts, and uncles may be dealing with cancer or another life-changing, life-threatening disease. You may be trying to deal with an emotional paralysis at the death of a loved one. You may feel you will never get past this, or that your life will never be the same. You can and will recover. But you won't be the same. However, it is not necessarily a bad thing. Why? That was the first question I asked God, myself, Daniel, and Dad. Why did this happen to you? Or, why NOT you?

You are meant to be where you are. Look around you. Challenges make us better. I will say it again. Yes, challenges make us better. What my mother went through was far more painful than I care to imagine. Caregivers become much stronger than they believe they can be.

If you lose someone to an illness, then you are the best advocate to help fight for a cure. You are the best person to help someone else who is going through what you have gone through. Who better to fight to cure Alzheimer's than me? I know what it takes to care for an Alzheimer's patient, so I should be the one out there fighting to make sure no one else has to go through that pain. That is how life works. We can either crawl into a hole or die or we can help make change.

I challenge you this! Find your photo album. Go ahead—I will wait. Now look at what you looked like when you were younger, before becoming a caregiver. If you are like me, I wore the craziest hairstyle any woman could wear and I just knew I looked good. Just find the picture of you. What were you thinking about at the time the picture was taken? I can almost guarantee it had nothing to do with caring for someone else, but here you are.

The difference between that picture and how you look today is that you lost your choices. That is why you need to fight back now. You need to get YOU back. Remember, caregivers forget who we are. We live so long for the next challenge, the next crisis, the next hospital visit, the next, the next, and the next. We forget about us.

Right now, go to the mirror. Turn the light on bright. Stare into that mirror. Look at you. What do you see? What do you want to see? In order to start healing, you will have to strip away the mask. Look at you. Think about what you have gone through. Do not move from that mirror until you really see yourself. You have aged. Some of us age faster than others. Stay there for as long as it takes you to realize who you are. You are a caregiver. You are stronger than you ever thought you would be. If you start to cry, then cry. Cry for as long as it takes. Because caregivers bundle up feelings for so long and never, allow ourselves to release the tears. It is painful. It is hard. It is not what you wanted to do. Stay there and observe the new you.

Now that the pity party is over, sit down. If you are like me, you are drained emotionally. I was exhausted when I did this and I did not know why. Now that I have thought about it, I realize that I finally allowed myself the time to grieve for me. Yes, the ME I lost. That is why I was crying. All those things I had planned for me are gone, and yet a new me has emerged. A better me.

If you are still a caregiver, each day, every day, look in a mirror and smile. Smile because you are you. You are a stronger person. You are what God made you to be. You are YOU and that is a good thing. We forget to give ourselves permission to be happy.

I give you permission to laugh. Once you accept you, you will be a better caregiver. You will not dread doing what you have to do. You will allow yourself to accept it. Now find one thing you used to do that you truly enjoyed. And DO it.

Many women go through the stages I did when I was young, but maybe not to the extreme I did. For years, each night I would plan what I was going to wear the next day and coordinate everything around it: hairstyle, purse, fingernail polish, earrings, watch—I changed watches every day—shoes, and dress or suit. That's what I did every night. Can you imagine how much energy it took me to do that every night!

So your challenge for tonight is this, before you go to bed, decide what outfit you are going to wear tomorrow. NO SWEATS! Paint your nails a different color (you know you can't afford and don't have the time to go to a nail shop). Pick up a book and read a chapter or just a paragraph. Do SOMETHING for yourself for just a little while. Before you go to bed, remember to smile in that mirror.

Remember, I have been there. Much of the time, I didn't care what I wore, be it fresh or not. Sweats were good enough. No makeup. Floppy shoes or tennis shoes, hair back, I grabbed my purse and that is how I presented myself for the day. Oh yes, I know what you look like. I was you. I challenge you to love yourself and care about YOU again.

About the Author

Marietta A. Harris was born in San Francisco CA. She is an accomplished musician, composer, motivational speaker, singer, and author. She has received numerous awards for outstanding work as an instructor and trainer. She currently resides in northern California.

This dynamic speaker now focuses her attention primarily on writing and motivational speaking. Her desire is to help others face their challenges and survive.

Her next book is scheduled for release in 2012.

Marietta A. Harris

<u>RESOURCES FOR YOU</u>

Alzheimer's Association

On Lok Senior Health

Social Services

Articles and Journals

Web MD

Alzheimer's Support Groups

Meals on Wheels

Senior Citizen Day Care

Your Physician

Your Spiritual Leader

Friends and Family

Support Groups—The Internet

Prayer